Nutrition in Pe

Editor

CORRI WOLF

PHYSICIAN ASSISTANT CLINICS

www.physicianassistant.theclinics.com

Consulting Editors
KIM ZUBER
JANE S. DAVIS

October 2022 • Volume 7 • Number 4

ELSEVIER

1600 John F. Kennedy Boulevard • Suite 1800 • Philadelphia, Pennsylvania, 19103-2899

http://www.theclinics.com

PHYSICIAN ASSISTANT CLINICS Volume 7, Number 4
October 2022 ISSN 2405-7991, ISBN-13: 978-0-323-96044-1

Editor: Taylor Hayes
Developmental Editor: Axell Ivan Jade Purificacion

Physician Assistant Clinics (ISSN: 2405–7991) is published quarterly by Elsevier Inc., 360 Park Avenue South, New York, NY 10010-1710. Months of issue are January, April, July, and October. Periodicals postage paid at New York, NY and additional mailing offices. Subscription prices are $150.00 per year (US individuals), $305.00 (US institutions), $100.00 (US students), $150.00 (Canadian individuals), $320.00 (Canadian institutions), $100.00 (Canadian students), $150.00 (international individuals), $320.00 (international institutions), and $100.00 (international students). Foreign air speed delivery is included in all *Clinics* subscription prices. All prices are subject to change without notice. POSTMASTER: Send address changes to *Physician Assistant Clinics*, Elsevier Periodicals Customer Service, 11830 Westline Industrial Drive, St. Louis, MO 63146. Customer Service Health Sciences Division, Subscription Customer Service, 3251 Riverport Lane, Maryland Heights, MO 63043. **Customer Service: 1-800-654-2452 (U.S. and Canada); 314-447-8871 (outside U.S. and Canada). Fax: 314-447-8029. E-mail: journalscustomerservice-usa@elsevier.com (for print support); journalsonlinesupport-usa@elsevier.com (for online support).**

Reprints. For copies of 100 or more, of articles in this publication, please contact the Commercial Reprints Department, Elsevier Inc., 360 Park Avenue South, New York, NY 10010-1710. Tel. 212-633-3874; Fax: 212-633-3820; E-mail: reprints@elsevier.com.

Physician Assistant Clinics is covered in *EMBASE/Excerpta Medica and ESCI.*

PROGRAM OBJECTIVE
The goal of the Physician Assistant Clinics is to keep practicing physician assistants up to date with current clinical practice by providing timely articles reviewing the state of the art in patient care.

TARGET AUDIENCE
Physician Assistants and other healthcare professionals

LEARNING OBJECTIVES
Upon completion of this activity, participants will be able to:
1. Review nutrition strategies for preventing chronic diseases, lowering the risk of obesity, morbidity, and mortality, and promoting nutrition.
2. Discuss the use of registered dieticians, nutritional, physical, and socioeconomic assessments, and evidence-based clinical guidelines as a holistic approach to nutritional care.
3. Recognize nutrition education and management as first-line therapies and preventative measures of chronic medical diseases, weight management, and injury throughout the lifespan.

ACCREDITATION
The Elsevier Office of Continuing Medical Education (EOCME) is accredited by the Accreditation Council for Continuing Medical Education (ACCME) to provide continuing medical education for physicians.

The EOCME designates this journal-based CME activity for a maximum of 13 *AMA PRA Category 1 Credit*(s)™. Physicians should claim only the credit commensurate with the extent of their participation in the activity.

All other health care professionals requesting continuing education credit for this enduring material will be issued a certificate of participation.

DISCLOSURE OF CONFLICTS OF INTEREST
The EOCME assesses conflict of interest with its instructors, faculty, planners, and other individuals who are in a position to control the content of CME activities. All relevant conflicts of interest that are identified are thoroughly vetted by EOCME for fair balance, scientific objectivity, and patient care recommendations. EOCME is committed to providing its learners with CME activities that promote improvements or quality in healthcare and not a specific proprietary business or a commercial interest.

The planning committee, staff, authors, and editors listed below have identified no financial relationships or relationships to products or devices they or their spouse/life partner have with commercial interest related to the content of this CME activity:
Teresa L. Armstead, MA, BS; Gabriela Barreto, MS, RD, CDN, CSSD; Melissa Bernstein, PhD, RDN, LD, FAND, DipACLM; Jay Bernstein, MD, MPH, MS, FACEP; Susan Ettinger, PhD, RD, DABN; Mindy Haar, PhD, RDN, CDN, FAND; Ahmad Hakemi, MD; Rachel Hercman, LCSW; Chelsea Jensen, MS, PA-C, RDN; Pradeep Kuttysankaran; Andrew Lundahl, PharmD; Mishaal Malik; Lorraine Laccetti Mongiello, Dr.PH, RDN, CDE; Elaina Osterbur, PhD; Erin L. Sherer, EdD, PA-C, RD; Jill R. Silverman, PhD, RDM; Tyler M. Simmons, ; Richard N. Steller, MD; Doreen Thomas-Payne, MSN, BSN, RN, PMHNP-BC; Christine Werner, PhD, PA-C, RDN; Corri Wolf, Ph.D., PA-C, RDN; Matthew Wright, MS, PA-C, RD

UNAPPROVED/OFF-LABEL USE DISCLOSURE
The EOCME requires CME faculty to disclose to the participants:
1. When products or procedures being discussed are off-label, unlabelled, experimental, and/or investigational (not US Food and Drug Administration [FDA] approved); and
2. Any limitations on the information presented, such as data that are preliminary or that represent ongoing research, interim analyses, and/or unsupported opinions. Faculty may discuss information about pharmaceutical agents that is outside of FDA-approved labelling. This information is intended solely for CME and is not intended to promote off-label use of these medications. If you have any questions, contact the medical affairs department of the manufacturer for the most recent prescribing information.

TO ENROLL
The CME program is available to all Physician Assistant Clinics subscribers at no additional fee. To subscribe to the Physician Assistant Clinics, call customer service at 1-800-654-2452 or sign up online at www.physicianassistant.theclinics.com.

METHOD OF PARTICIPATION

In order to claim credit, participants must complete the following:

1. Complete enrolment as indicated above
2. Read the activity
3. Complete the CME Test and Evaluation. Participants must achieve a score of 70% on the test. All CME Tests and Evaluations must be completed online

CME INQUIRIES/SPECIAL NEEDS

For all CME inquiries or special needs, please contact elsevierCME@elsevier.com.

Contributors

CONSULTING EDITORS

KIM ZUBER, PAC, MS
Executive Director, American Academy of Nephrology PAs, St Petersburg, Florida

JANE S. DAVIS, DNP
Division of Nephrology, The University of Alabama at Birmingham, Birmingham, Alabama

EDITOR

CORRI WOLF, PhD, PA-C, RDN
Associate Professor, Department of Physician Assistant Studies, Assistant Dean, School of Health Professions, New York Institute of Technology, Old Westbury, New York

AUTHORS

TERESA L. ARMSTEAD, MA, BS
Executive Secretary, Central Michigan University Physician Assistant Program, Mount Pleasant, Michigan

GABRIELA BARRETO, MS, RD, CDN, CSSD
Professor of Nutrition, St. Joseph's College, Brooklyn, New York

JAY BERNSTEIN, MD, MPH, MS, FACEP
Assistant Professor, Clerkship Director, Department of Emergency Medicine, Boonshoft School of Medicine, Wright State University, Fairborn, Ohio

MELISSA BERNSTEIN, PhD, RDN, LD, FAND, DipACLM
Associate Professor and Chair, Department of Nutrition, Rosalind Franklin University of Medicine and Science, North Chicago, Illinois

SUSAN ETTINGER, PhD, RD, DABN
Adjunct Associate Professor, New York Institute of Technology, Research Associate, Mount Sinai Morningside Hospital Center, New York, New York

MINDY HAAR, PhD, RDN, CDN, FAND
Clinical Associate Professor, Chair, Department of Interdisciplinary Health Sciences, Assist Dean, Undergraduate Affairs, School of Health Professions, New York Institute of Technology, Old Westbury, New York

AHMAD HAKEMI, MD
Medical Director, Central Michigan University Physician Assistant Program, Mount Pleasant, Michigan

RACHEL HERCMAN, LCSW
Psychotherapist in Private Practice, New York, New York

CHELSEA JENSEN, MS, PA-C, RDN
Department of Neurosurgery, Neuroscience ICU, Northwell Health South Shore University Hospital, Bay Shore, New York

LORRAINE LACCETTI MONGIELLO, DrPH, RDN, CDE
Associate Professor, Clinical Nutrition and Interdisciplinary Health Sciences, New York Institute of Technology, Old Westbury, New York

ANDREW LUNDAHL, PharmD
Clinical Pharmacist, Mission Pharmacy, Mount Pleasant, Michigan

MISHAAL MALIK, BS
Medical School Student, Central Michigan University, Mount Pleasant, Michigan

ELAINA OSTERBUR, PhD
Program in Health Sciences, Department of Clinical Health Sciences, Associate Professor, Saint Louis University, DCHS, St Louis, Missouri

ERIN L. SHERER, EdD, PA-C, RD
Emergency Department, Columbia University Irving Medical Center, New York, New York

JILL R. SILVERMAN, PhD, RDN
Assistant Professor, Department of Nutrition Science, Farmingdale State College, Farmingdale, New York

TYLER M. SIMMONS, BS
Physician Assistant Student, Central Michigan University, Mount Pleasant, Michigan

RICHARD N. STELLER, MD
Gastroenterology, Medical Director, Catholic Health Physician Partners at Merrick, Merrick, New York

CHRISTINE WERNER, PhD, PA-C, RDN
Physician Assistant Program, Department of Clinical Health Sciences, Professor, Saint Louis University, DCHS, St Louis, Missouri

CORRI WOLF, PhD, PA-C, RDN
Associate Professor, Department of Physician Assistant Studies, Assistant Dean, School of Health Professions, New York Institute of Technology, Old Westbury, New York

MATTHEW WRIGHT, MS, PA-C, RD
Lecturer, Physician Assistant Studies and Practice, Rutgers University, School of Health Profession, Piscataway, New Jersey

Contents

Nutrition interventions are critical components of preventative care and chronic disease management. However, data exist demonstrating a lack of comfort in addressing nutrition-related concerns as well as in conducting nutrition assessments on the part of a variety of medical providers. Nutrition history assessments such as the 24-h dietary recall, food journal, and food frequency questionnaires (FFQs) allow providers to assess a patient's recent dietary intake and subsequently deliver individualized dietary counseling. When combined with a standard physical examination focused on pathology potentially related to nutritional causes, providers will gain considerable insight into nutrition-related contributions to risk and disease states. The current article will review nutrition-assessment tools and physical examination findings associated with nutrient deficiencies and make recommendations as to how these may be incorporated into a busy medical practice.

Obesity rates are increasing in the United States while evidence continues to support its relationship to chronic disease. Health-care professionals often approach the discussion of weight with judgment, further alienating patients from getting the care they need. Many factors affect patient weight and include physiologic, psychological, environmental, economic influences as well as nutrition literacy. Providers may optimize chances for patient lifestyle change when they examine their own biases, moderate their language, attend to their nonverbal communication, use motivational interviewing, emphasize the impact of small but sustainable changes, consider individualized approaches, and include nutrition professionals as part of the health-care team.

Following a healthy dietary pattern throughout the lifespan is vital to achieving and maintaining good health and reducing the risk of chronic disease. Nutrition is the first line of treatment and prevention of commonly encountered medical conditions and patients often seek nutrition advice from their medical providers, which underscores the need for knowledge in this area. To provide effective nutrition counseling, a clinician must have a solid understanding of nutrients. This article introduces the macronutrients: carbohydrate, protein, and fat and their association with commonly encountered gastrointestinal disorders.

A healthy diet is recognized as important for overall well-being. Besides the increase in lifespan, a healthy diet lowers the risk of certain types of cancers, obesity, type 2 diabetes, cardiovascular disease, and stroke. Plant-based diets are considered safe and nutritious; however, certain nutrients may be lacking in plant sources. Therefore, careful meal planning is required to ensure the intake of the recommended dietary allowances of nutrients. The Mediterranean diet, Paleo diet, and intermittent fasting are a few types of diets that confer specific health benefits when adopted with appropriate planning.

Cardiovascular disease (CVD) is a leading cause of morbidity and mortality worldwide; poor diet is a contributing factor to the development of CVD. Recent nutritional guidance for CVD prevention focuses on life-long healthy dietary patterns. Evidence-based dietary patterns encourage high intakes of vegetables, fruits, plant-based proteins (beans and legumes), and whole grains. Food sources higher in saturated fat, trans fat, cholesterol, added sugar, and sodium should be limited within the diet. Clinicians should understand current dietary guidelines to support research-centered discussions about nutrition with patients. Registered dietitians are a valuable source for clinicians and patients seeking assistance understanding nutrition guidelines.

Although research has not identified one ideal diet for all those with diabetes, it does provide overwhelming evidence that food choices and eating patterns will affect glycemia, health goals, and quality of life. Therefore, meal planning must be individualized for each patient considering their health status, resources, personal preferences, motivation, and glycemic targets. Although the Registered Dietitian/Nutritionist is the primary provider of nutrition counseling and education, it is essential that all members of the health care team are equipped to counter the barrage of deceptive and often dangerous nutrition information that their patients receive from social media and elsewhere.

Carbohydrate counting, both basic and advanced, is an effective and rec-ommended meal-planning strategy to achieve glycemic targets in persons with both type 1 and type 2 diabetes. They empower patients by allowing freedom of food choices and greater mealtime flexibility. Whereas these methods ultimately simplify food decisions, initially they can be daunting. Therefore, it is necessary that primary care providers understand these methods to provide ongoing education and support to their patients. This primer explains how carbohydrates, protien, and fat affect blood glucose and how to determine "carb allowances" and pre-meal basal insu-lin doses.

The diet industry accrued >$71 billion in 2020, yet over 42% of American adults have obesity, a chronic disease state associated with type 2 dia-betes, coronary vascular disease, and sleep apnea. With a reported 80–95% of people regaining weight loss through diet and exercise alone, it is important to consider alternative strategies for sustainable weight loss. Bariatric surgeries result in maintainable weight loss due to a signif-icant reduction in food intake and inhibition of energy absorption. Howev-er, continued success requires a lifetime commitment to behavior modification and dietary compliance.

Chronic kidney disease (CKD) is increasing rapidly against a background of widespread obesity, diabetes, chronic inflammation, and oxidative stress. Metabolic diseases trigger aberrant metabolic pathways that inten-sify gut dysbiosis and increase the likelihood that the kidney will be damaged and inexorably progress to end-stage kidney disease (ESKD). Abundant literature supports the role of diet in preventing and controlling the extent of kidney damage. This review will discuss evidence that sup-ports the role of selected diet strategies for patients with CKD. These stra-tegies have the potential to reduce initial kidney damage and slow progression to ESKD.

Critical illness causes several metabolic changes, many of which affect nutritional status. Numerous studies demonstrate that providing adequate nutrition during critical illness improves patient outcomes and overall re-covery. Most patients will benefit from enteral over parenteral nutrition. Although there may be barriers to providing nutrition, such as diarrhea or risk of aspiration, continued nutrition support is recommended. Specific disease states have varying nutrition recommendations, but most impor-tant is providing early (within 24–48 hours) and adequate (>80% energy and protein needs) nutrition to aid in healing.

> A high-quality, nutritious diet is essential to optimize health and well-being at any age. A poor-quality diet can result in inadequate intake of energy and essential nutrients, resulting in malnutrition and worsening of physical and mental health status. Selection of nutritious foods to meet individual nutrient needs is therefore increasingly important with age. Efforts to consume a nutritious diet can be influenced by health status and factors that may occur naturally with aging, or as a result of illness. Individualized guidance should be designed to help overcome medical, physical, economic, and social barriers to eating a healthy diet.

> Athletes have unique energy and nutrients to compensate for their high energy output and demands on their bodies to optimize performance and health. Of most importance is ensuring adequate energy intake to enhance performance, minimize injury risk, and avoid low energy availability. The consequences of poor nutrition in athletes can lead to increased risk of injury, suboptimal performance, and Relative Energy Deficiency in Sport. This can be achieved through a nutrition plan that emphasizes adequate protein, carbohydrates, fat, hydration, and supplements with specific nutrient timing.

> Athletes train and perform at intense activity levels and have specific nutrient requirements. Their energy needs are often double their metabolism. Hence, they accordingly require tailored nutrition plans. During injury recovery, supplementation along with protein intake can be advantageous. Athletes are also prone to factors, such as low energy availability, disordered eating, and eating disorders, which can impact metabolic, cardiac, skeletal, reproductive, and mental health as well as performance. In this article, we discuss the nutrition recommendations regarding supplementation, injury recovery, relative energy deficiency, and eating disorders in athletes.

PHYSICIAN ASSISTANT CLINICS

FORTHCOMING ISSUES

January 2023
Emergency Medicine
Dan Tzizik, *Editor*

April 2023
Pharmacology
Rebecca Maxson, *Editor*

July 2023
Emerging and Re-Emerging Infectious Diseases
Gerald Kayingo, *Editor*

RECENT ISSUES

July 2022
Obstetrics and Gynecology
Elyse Watkins, *Editor*

April 2022
The Kidney
Kim Zuber and Jane Davis, *Editors*

January 2022
Preventive Medicine
Stephanie Neary, *Editor*

SERIES OF RELATED INTEREST

Primary Care: Clinics in Office Practice
https://www.primarycare.theclinics.com/

THE CLINICS ARE AVAILABLE ONLINE!
Access your subscription at:
www.theclinics.com

Foreword

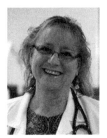 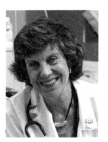

Kim Zuber, PAC, MS Jane S. Davis, DNP
Consulting Editors

Food. The word figures often in our conversations and our literature. There is food for thought, bread is the staff of life, food coma, "quite a dish" for the beautiful male/female, butterfingers, humble pie, big cheese; the list is endless. Nutrition as part of treatment is not limited to the care of patients with diabetes or cardiac issues. Rather, it is a part of caring for patients across disciplines and disease states.

Wolf and an outstanding collection of authors have created a manual for nutrition education that will be valuable to anyone in medicine. This will be the go-to source for anyone who has approached the sensitive topic of weight loss with a patient or family member as well as managed patients in the intensive care units requiring parental nutrition. And everything in between.

The Internet, social media, and print publications abound with fad diets, food tips, and the ever-present ads touting how eating some food will add years to life. Steering patients away from these false promises is challenging but possible. It depends on the approach.

"You are what you eat" affects many aspects of health. With this issue of *Physician Assistant Clinics*, the seasoned PA as well as the inexperienced student will find

Physician Assist Clin 7 (2022) xiii–xiv
https://doi.org/10.1016/j.cpha.2022.08.002
2405-7991/22/© 2022 Published by Elsevier Inc.

physicianassistant.theclinics.com

valuable information to enhance and inform their practice. We hope you enjoy it as much as we did, and, more importantly, find it useful in your practices.

Kim Zuber, PAC, MS
American Academy of Nephrology Pas
131 31st Avenue North
St Petersburg, FL 33704, USA

Jane S. Davis, DNP
University of Alabama at Birmingham
728 Richard Arrington Boulevard South
Birmingham, AL 35233, USA

E-mail addresses:
zuberkim@yahoo.com (K. Zuber, PAC)
jsdavis@uabmc.edu (J.S. Davis)

Preface

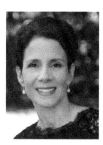

Corri Wolf, PhD, PA-C, RDN
Editor

Welcome to *Physician Assistant Clinics*, Nutrition in Patient Care. Nutrition has been touched upon in previous issues as it related to specific topics. However, this issue is dedicated specifically to nutrition. This is an exciting opportunity because evidence confirms the central role nutrition plays in preventing and managing major causes of mortality and morbidity. Despite its role in patient care and chronic disease, many physician assistant (PA) programs and conferences provide few if any offerings devoted to diet and nutrition. To provide optimal care, regardless of practice area, PAs must have a sound foundation in nutrition, and this issue promises to fill knowledge gaps.

This *Physician Assistant Clinics* issue encompasses a broad range of nutrition topics, including the first step to patient care: nutrition assessment. Wright teaches the reader how to take a nutrition-focused history and incorporate a nutrition-focused physical exam into everyday practice. Haar and Hercman highlight the often-awkward topic of discussing weight with patients while reviewing the prevalence of obesity and overweight with its subsequent effects on health outcomes. The October 2021 issue focused on gastroenterology and stressed the need to provide a solid foundation in the nutrients. Wolf and Steller take a deeper dive into the nutrients and their association with common gastrointestinal disorders.

Every day, new diets are being promoted on the Internet and through social media, and patients look to PAs for guidance. Werner and Osterbur have an article dedicated to decoding plant-based and other popular diets to help PAs confidently answer patients' questions while ensuring they are meeting their nutrient needs.

The relationship between diet, disease, and nutrition is the first line of treatment and prevention for a multitude of chronic conditions. Included are articles on nutrition and cardiovascular disease by Sherer, Hakemi, Lundahl, Armstread, Malik, and Simmons. Nutrition and diabetes is addressed by Mongiello and includes carbohydrate counting and obesity. Then, Silverman teaches us postoperative nutritional management after bariatric surgery, and Ettinger discusses diet strategies for the patient with chronic kidney disease. Jensen, Bernstein, and Bernstein cover nutritional health for special

Physician Assist Clin 7 (2022) xv–xvi
https://doi.org/10.1016/j.cpha.2022.08.001
2405-7991/22/ **physicianassistant.theclinics.com**

populations, including the older adult and the critically ill patient. Last, Barreto provides an evidenced-based review on sports nutrition and, for those PAs who work with athletes or aspire to be one themselves, this issue includes a deeper dive that goes beyond the basics.

Our sincere hope is that readers will better understand their patients' nutritional needs and apply what they learn from these evidence-based review articles to their everyday practice. Furthermore, we hope this issue will be used as assigned reading for PA students as they progress through their didactic education and supervised clinical practice experiences.

Corri Wolf, PhD, PA-C, RDN
Department of Physician Assistant Studies
School of Health Professions
New York Institute of Technology
Old Westbury, NY 11568, USA

E-mail address:
cwolf01@nyit.edu

Nutrition Assessment
Nutrition-Focused History and Physical Examination

Matthew Wright, MS, PA-C, RD

KEYWORDS

- Nutrition assessment • 24-hour recall • Food frequency questionnaire
- Nutrition-focused physical examination

KEY POINTS

- Nutrition is a critical component of preventative care and chronic disease management.
- Nutrition-related assessments have the potential to significantly improve chronic disease management.
- Opportunities exist to further implement nutrition histories and screenings in medical practice.
- Nutrition history screening tools include the 24-h recall, food journals, and food frequency questionnaires (FFQs).
- Nutrition-focused physical examination should be combined with nutrition history screening tools.

INTRODUCTION

Nutrition is a critical component of preventive medicine and chronic disease management.[1,2] Nutritional interventions in both capacities are essential for health care providers to understand and implement effectively. Previous cross-sectional survey data from Hanson and colleagues[3] have demonstrated that clinically working physician assistants (PA) in various fields routinely encounter patients with nutrition-related medical diagnoses. However, only 25% of respondents reported feeling "very confident" in their ability to address nutrition-related concerns or create a nutrition management plan. Further, 27% reported being "not comfortable" in addressing nutrition-related concerns.[3] Similar findings were demonstrated in a sample of PA students from a single Midwestern PA program. Survey results of students in the clinical phase of their program showed that only half of respondents expressed a moderate level of confidence in designing a nutritional plan based on a medical diagnosis, and 100% of respondents felt they needed additional education in lifestyle management.[4]

Physician Assistant Studies and Practice Rutgers University, School of Health Professions, 675 Hoes Lane West, 6th Floor, Piscataway, NJ 08854, USA
E-mail address: wrightmj@shp.rutgers.edu

Physician Assist Clin 7 (2022) 579–587
https://doi.org/10.1016/j.cpha.2022.05.001
2405-7991/22/© 2022 Elsevier Inc. All rights reserved.

Medical students, residents, and physicians have previously reported deficiencies in nutrition knowledge [5,6], and similar findings have been identified in medical school curriculums.[7] Thematic analyses of qualitative focus group interviews with medical students demonstrated the emergence of themes involving minimal integration of nutrition into the medical curriculum and a lack of observed nutrition counseling by shadowed physicians. Further, residents reported frustration at their lack of nutrition knowledge for lifestyle counseling.[5] Previous quantitative data have demonstrated similar findings in a cross-sectional analysis of dietary counseling during internal medicine residencies.[6] Of the 40 internal medicine residency program directors and the 133 residents who participated in the study, survey results demonstrated that less than 50% of the program directors provided "extensive or quite a bit of" training in dietary counseling, and less than 10% of residents received a formal nutrition education curriculum. Among the barriers found to counseling, lower faculty nutrition expertise was noted to be related to reduced educational offerings for residents.[6]

Nursing faculty in the United States involved in training nurse practitioners (NPs) and doctors of nursing practice have also documented deficiencies in nutrition education. In a cross-sectional study of faculty from primary care NP programs, the mean hours of nutrition education were 14.4 across 49 schools. Of all respondents, only 39% felt their students received adequate training in nutrition, and 75.6% thought it was very or extremely important to become more educated about nutrition.[8]

Dietary counseling, including individualized diet assessment and intervention delivered by dietitians, has been proven to be of significant benefit. When compared with usual care or minimal dietary counseling, individualized assessment and recommendations have led to significant reductions in body weight, waist circumference, and measures of glycemia in the primary care patient population.[9] Given that 860 million annual adult visits to ambulatory medical offices occurred in 2018 alone,[10] an abundance of opportunity exists for individualized dietary assessment and counseling to be delivered by medical providers.

Considering this ample opportunity, the purpose of the current review article is to describe the utility of current subjective and objective nutrition assessments and describe how each may be incorporated into the daily practice of medical care providers.

TOOLS FOR THE ASSESSMENT OF NUTRITIONAL INTAKE
24-Hour Dietary Recall and Food Records

The 24-h dietary recall is a widely used screening tool to assess nutrient intake in both nutritional epidemiology studies and clinical practice. Practitioners obtain retrospective, historical information by asking a series of dietary questions designed to assess all food and drink consumed over an entire 24-h period. Questions included in the 24-h recall are food characteristics (frozen, canned, fresh, preserved, and so forth), cooking method (fried, baked, grilled, and so forth), amount consumed, and additives such as condiments, sauces, and dressings. Additionally, assessments of the timing of meals and location are included in the inquiry.[11]

The accuracy of information obtained depends on both the interviewer's skills and the patient's memory. Castell and colleagues have previously discussed several advantages and disadvantages.[11] Noted disadvantages of the 24-h recall potentially affecting its utilization and accuracy include the practitioner's knowledge of food portions and calorie estimation, limitations of patient's memory, and 24 hours may not be reflective of usual intake.[11] However, several limitations can be mitigated by using the United States Department of Agriculture's (USDA) multi-pass method,[12] as well as further dietary continuing education for medical providers.

The most pertinent advantages applying directly to a medical practice include the rapidity of completion and the high precision with which information can be collected.[11] However, perhaps of most importance, the 24-h recall has been demonstrated to be reliable and valid in a wide variety of patients in regard to total energy intake[12,13] and may be a suitable screening for intake of individual nutrients such as sodium.[14]

Further, if desired to save time, a 24-h dietary recall can be self-collected by the patient in advance of an appointment for clinician review. Evidence has previously demonstrated the effectiveness of online, self-reported 24-h recalls.[15] However, the collection of multiple days may be necessary to increase the potential for the representation of usual eating habits and accuracy in estimates of calorie intake.[16] This procedure represents a patient collected food record, or food journal, frequently involving 3 to 5-day intervals, but can be an additional patient recording burden. Repeated measures have the potential to improve accuracy with clinical or self-reporting assessments.

In clinical practice, the accuracy of the 24-h recall is enhanced with the multi-pass method (**Table 1**). As previously described by the USDA, the multi-pass method follows a five-step approach. Initially, step 1 involves providers obtaining a "quick list" of all foods and beverages consumed the previous day, beginning from the first item consumed from the time of awakening to the last consumed at the end of the day. In step 2, the provider will review the list obtained and ask about potential forgotten foods. In step 3, time and occasion are recorded for everything consumed, and in step 4, descriptions and amounts are collected. Inquiring about portions in step 4 should be conducted using relatable points of reference patients will understand that roughly estimate standard portion sizes as described in **Table 2**. Finally, step 5 involves a final recheck for any missing foods.[17] Following a thorough nutrition history, individualized nutrition interventions based on the patient's comorbidities or pertinent risk factors can be implemented.

Food Frequency Questionnaires

Food frequency questionnaires (FFQ) are an alternative assessment to the 24-h recall and the extended food record. Utilization involves patients noting the frequency with which they consume representative foods from the major food groups within specific periods of time.[19] The FFQ is a versatile tool capable of being adapted based on the nutrients of concern for specific disease states and has previously been conducted for dietary screening in cardiovascular disease prevention.[20] Given the capacity to identify

Table 1 USDA 5-pass method for obtaining a 24-hour recall	
Step	**Description**
Step 1 (first pass)	Quick list of all foods and beverages for each meal and snack consumed.
Step 2 (second pass)	Review quick list. Ask about forgotten foods (eg, condiments, sauces, dressings, candies, or other sweets).
Step 3 (third pass)	Record the time of all food recorded and occasion (eg, breakfast, lunch, dinner, snack).
Step 4 (fourth pass)	Descriptions of foods (grilled, baked, fried, broiled, and so forth). Amounts consumed (1/2 cup, 1 bowl, 1 glass, and so forth).
Step 5 (fifth and final pass)	Similar to step 2, final screening for missing foods.

Information in tablet from reference.[17]

Table 2 Common portion size estimators[18]	
Portion Size Estimator	**Food Serving**
Palm of hand = 3oz	Meat, fish, poultry such as chicken or turkey breast
1 Fist or tennis ball or baseball = 1 cup	Salad, mashed potatoes, ice cream, 1 medium-sized fruit such as apple, orange, peach, pear, and so forth
Size of thumb (tip to base) = 1 ounce	Cheese, meats
Tip of thumb = teaspoon	Butter (1 pad)

food patterns, clinicians are provided the ability to identify risk factors in their patient's usual eating habits and deliver individualized counseling beyond a retrospective 24-h. Additional advantages include reduced time burden in obtaining information for clinicians and a lower skill level in interpreting and collecting data. However, consideration should be given to several disadvantages. FFQs have the propensity to overestimate specific food groups, particularly those which may be under-consumed such as vegetables. Further, not all FFQs incorporate measurement of dietary intakeas quantities of specific foods are not generally obtained.[19] A thorough understanding of the information collected and the limitations of assessment method are necessary when selecting a specific tool to measure the individualized dietary intakes of patients.

OBJECTIVE ASSESSMENT OF NUTRITIONAL STATUS
Nutrition-Focused Physical Examination

A wide variety of physical findings from the standard office-based physical examination provide insight into a patient's nutrition status. In collaboration, the American Academy of Nutrition and Dietetics (AAND) and the American Society for Parenteral and Enteral Nutrition (ASPEN) developed an objective definition for malnutrition reflecting findings documented during physical examination (**Table 3**). Along with reduced energy intake and weight loss, loss of muscle mass and subcutaneous fat, local or generalized edema, and reduced functional status typically measured by hand-grip strength make up the criteria on which malnutrition is based. Two positive findings documented from the physical examination and nutrition history diagnose malnutrition.[21] Longitudinal weight loss ranging from acute periods of weeks to chronic periods up to 1-year should be expressed as percent loss from a patient's typical baseline to establish the weight loss criteria in the diagnosis of malnutrition. Body mass index (BMI) will decline with persistent weight loss, though providers should be aware that BMI does not need to indicate underweight classification to establish malnutrition or a malnourished state.[21]

Table 3 AAND/ASPEN criteria for malnutrition and signs on physical examination	
Malnutrition Criteria[a]	**Physical Examination Finding**
Loss of subcutaneous fat	Fat loss in areas of triceps, orbits, over ribs, weight trend
Loss of muscle	Temporalis muscle wasting, clavicular pitting, pectoral and deltoid wasting, scapular, quadriceps, and gastrocnemius wasting, weight trend
Fluid accumulation	Generalized or localized edema
Hand grip strength	Hand dynamometer strength

Criteria in table from reference.[21]
[a] Additional criteria not found with physical examination: reduced nutritional consumption.

Identifying the signs and symptoms indicative of malnutrition are particularly important for hospitalized and surgical populations. Malnutrition has been identified as an independent risk factor for increased morbidity and mortality in the postoperative period and increased hospital length of stay.[22] Risks are compounded by the high likelihood of the presence of malnourishment before elective surgery, with a particular burden on those undergoing oncologic and gastroenterological procedures.[23] Greater identification of malnourishment using tools of diet analyses and a thorough nutrition-related physical examination offers the possibility to identify preprocedural risk and intervene to reduce surgical complications.

Along with calories and macronutrients, cues to micronutrient deficiency may also be identified with a thorough physical examination. Findings may further be reinforced when combined with the utilization of a dietary assessment tool. Common signs and symptoms indicative of potential micronutrient deficiencies are found in **Table 4** and should be identified systematically. Alternations in the color and integrity of skin and mucosal surfaces may represent findings indicative of micronutrient deficiencies, as well as other findings in the ocular, oral, musculoskeletal, and neurologic systems.[24] Particular attention should be paid to patients with conditions potentially causing gastrointestinal malabsorption or those leading to restrictions in intake. Common comorbid-medical disorders contributing to deficiency syndromes include alcoholism, inflammatory bowel diseases, pancreatic insufficiency, celiac disease, bariatric surgery, congestive heart failure, and diabetes.[24-26] Additionally, lower socioeconomic status should be considered a risk factor, and patients with limited capacity to access nutrient-dense foods should be provided additional screening.[27]

DISCUSSION

Standard office-based assessments, as described above, offer considerable potential for thorough nutrition screening and monitoring. Obtaining a nutrition history such as a 24-h recall or an FFQ allows medical providers to gain insight into eating habits and

Table 4
Nutrition-focused physical examination findings of micronutrient deficiencies

Body System	Finding and Associated Nutrient(s) Deficiency, Toxicity
Skin/oral mucosa	Mucosal pallor: iron, B12, folic acid, copper deficiency Yellowing of skin: vitamin A toxicity Dermatitis: riboflavin, niacin, vitamin B6, biotin deficiency Petechiae, bruising, gum bleeding: vitamin K, vitamin C deficiencies Poor wound healing: zinc, vitamin C deficiencies
Nails	Spoon-nails: iron deficiency Brittle nails: biotin deficiency
Hair	Corkscrew hair, coiled hair: vitamin C deficiency Brittle hair, alopecia: biotin
Eyes	Conjunctival pallor: iron, B12, folic acid deficiency Dryness, white lesions: vitamin A deficiency Ophthalmoplegia: thiamine deficiency
Musculoskeletal	Softening of long bones, bow legs (osteomalacia): vitamin D deficiency Increased fracture incidence: calcium deficiency Swollen joints, joint pain: vitamin C, vitamin D deficiency
Neurologic	Ataxia, confusion: thiamine deficiency Tremors, seizures: calcium deficiency

Data in table from references.[24-26]

patterns that may contribute to chronic disease development or progression.[28,29] Additionally, nutrition histories may allow for adequate estimation of micronutrient intakes[14] and, when combined with a nutrition-focused physical examination, can aid in identifying deficiencies.[24,26] Using office-based tools in regular practice offers the possibility to provide individualized dietary recommendations based specifically on current habits.

As briefly mentioned, nutrition counseling and lifestyle interventions play critical roles in disease prevention. A recent systematic review and meta-analysis[30] of randomized-controlled trials conducted in patients with impaired fasting glucose and dyslipidemia demonstrated the effectiveness of nutrition in the prevention of progression to diabetes. Among 7 randomized-controlled trials, a risk reduction of 0.53 (CI: 0.41–0.67) was noted with lifestyle interventions targeted for weight loss, increased physical activity, higher fiber, and a low saturated fat diet.[30] However, it should be noted that evidence was less strong across trials for the prevention of secondary complications, perhaps indicating nutrition screenings with diet histories should begin in early adulthood when morbidity burden is relatively less frequent.

Similar evidence has been demonstrated in primary and secondary cardiovascular disease prevention in a meta-analysis of 30 randomized controlled trials,[31] all exploring the benefits of following a Mediterranean Diet pattern. Interestingly, across studies, only small-to-modest evidence supported reductions in total cholesterol, and moderate evidence supported reductions in systolic and diastolic blood pressure. Additionally, it was mainly determined to be low-quality evidence on reductions in LDL cholesterol and triglycerides. Similar quality evidence was noted for reductions in cardiovascular mortality and total mortality.[31] Despite the lower quality of evidence, the cumulative evidence for nutritional interventions in cardiovascular disease did lead to improvement in risk factors for heart disease.

These findings are reinforced by separate work on common diets designed to manipulate macronutrient distributions for weight loss, such as low-to moderate-carbohydrate diets and low-fat diets.[32] Along with weight loss, outcomes in this systematic macronutrient review included cholesterol levels, blood pressure, and c-reactive protein levels. Cumulatively, low and moderate carbohydrate diets demonstrated significant reductions in weight, total and LDL cholesterol, and blood pressure readings. Additionally, the Dietary Approaches to Stop Hypertension (DASH) diet demonstrated similar weight and blood pressure reductions.[32] These findings add further evidence and reinforce findings on the Mediterranean Diet pattern demonstrating the effectiveness of nutrition interventions for mitigating predisposing factors of chronic disease.

Given the noted benefit of nutrition interventions, screening and personalized recommendations have the potential to significantly impact patient care by reducing morbidity. Medical providers have a significant opportunity to gain further knowledge of nutrition therapies and use tools to individualize counseling. While a busy medical office affords little time for additional counseling and nutrition management, obtaining nutrition-histories are relatively quick procedures designed to empower providers with additional insight into their patient's lifestyle . Further, additional knowledge of dietary contributions to disease risk and chronic disease management may facilitate a greater frequency of referrals to registered dietitians, the nutrition experts on the interdisciplinary health care team.

SUMMARY

Opportunities exist to conduct nutrition histories at appointments designed for follow-up on medication and disease management and at annual well-visits by reviewing patient-collected food journals. Further, the FFQ may be designed for specific medical specialties for brief screenings in the office to identify dietary patterns placing patients at additional risk for disease or secondary complications. Additionally, for certain patients, providers may wish to establish appointments specifically designed to collect a 24-h recall and provide brief, individualized screening, and counseling. Identifying nutrition concerns with screening and assessment may facilitate more frequent referrals to registered dietitians for expert nutritional support as evidence consistently demonstrates their efficacy in improving clinical parameters of chronic disease.[33,34] Significant consideration should be given to incorporating a nutrition-screening tool along with a thorough nutrition-focused examination into routine practice and increased frequency of dietitian referral when nutrition-related concerns are identified.

CLINICS CARE POINTS

- Nutrition screening and assessment allow for the identification of food-related factors potentially contributing to disease risk and control.
- A thorough understanding of patients' nutritional habits provides important information to facilitate beneficial lifestyle counseling and referral.
- Various screening tools exist for nutrition assessment to be readily incorporated into clinical practice.
- Nutrition screening and intervention contribute significantly to patient care outcomes.
- Referral to a dietitian is highly beneficial for disease prevention and as an additional measure to promote disease management.

DISCLOSURE

The author has nothing to disclose.

REFERENCES

1. Becerra-Tomás N, Blanco Mejía S, Viguiliouk E, et al. Mediterranean diet, cardiovascular disease and mortality in diabetes: A systematic review and meta-analysis of prospective cohort studies and randomized clinical trials. Crit Rev Food Sci Nutr 2020;60(7):1207–27.
2. Rosato V, Temple NJ, La Vecchia C, et al. Mediterranean diet and cardiovascular disease: a systematic review and meta-analysis of observational studies. Eur J Nutr 2019;58(1):173–91.
3. Hanson CK, Woscyna G, Jensen SK, et al. Demographics and nutrition-related patient care encounters: a survey of physician assistants in Nebraska. J Physician Assist Educ 2013;24(3):6–13.
4. Abreu A, Keyes SK, Faries MD. Physician Assistant Students' Perceptions and Competencies Concerning Lifestyle Medicine. J Physician Assist Educ 2021; 32(2):97–101.
5. Danek RL, Berlin KL, Waite GN, et al. Perceptions of Nutrition Education in the Current Medical School Curriculum. Fam Med 2017;49(10):803–6.
6. Khandelwal S, Zemore SE, Hemmerling A. Nutrition Education in Internal Medicine Residency Programs and Predictors of Residents' Dietary Counseling Practices. J Med Educ Curric Dev 2018;5. 2382120518763360.

7. Crowley J, Ball L, Hiddink GJ. Nutrition in medical education: a systematic review. Lancet Planet Health 2019;3(9):e379–89.

8. Chao AM, Zhou Y, Wei X, et al. Nutrition Education in Primary Care Adult and Family Nurse Practitioner Programs. Nurse Educ 2022;47(1):47–50.

9. Mitchell LJ, Ball LE, Ross LJ, et al. Effectiveness of Dietetic Consultations in Primary Health Care: A Systematic Review of Randomized Controlled Trials. J Acad Nutr Diet 2017;117(12):1941–62.

10. CDC. Ambulatory care use and physician office visits. Available at: https://www.cdc.gov/nchs/fastats/physician-visits.htm. Accessed March 9, 2021.

11. Salvador Castell G, Serra-Majem L, Ribas-Barba L. What and how much do we eat? 24-hour dietary recall method. Nutr Hosp 2015;31(Suppl 3):46–8.

12. Conway JM, Ingwersen LA, Moshfegh AJ. Accuracy of dietary recall using the USDA five-step multiple-pass method in men: an observational validation study. J Am Diet Assoc 2004;104(4):595–603.

13. Ard JD, Desmond RA, Allison DB, et al. Dietary restraint and disinhibition do not affect accuracy of 24-hour recall in a multiethnic population. J Am Diet Assoc 2006;106(3):434–7.

14. McLean R, Cameron C, Butcher E, et al. Comparison of 24-hour urine and 24-hour diet recall for estimating dietary sodium intake in populations: A systematic review and meta-analysis. J Clin Hypertens (Greenwich) 2019;21(12):1753–62.

15. Foster E, Lee C, Imamura F, et al. Validity and reliability of an online self-report 24-h dietary recall method (Intake24): a doubly labelled water study and repeated-measures analysis. J Nutr Sci 2019;8:e29.

16. Jackson KA, Byrne NM, Magarey AM, et al. Minimizing random error in dietary intakes assessed by 24-h recall, in overweight and obese adults. Eur J Clin Nutr 2008;62(4):537–43.

17. Raper NPB, Ingwersen L, Steinfeldt L, et al. An overview of USDA's dietary intake data system. J Food Compost Anal 2004;17(3–4):545–55.

18. Diabetes Meal Planning. cdc.gov. Updated March 11, 2021. https://www.cdc.gov/diabetes/managing/eat-well/meal-plan-method.html. Accessed June 30, 2022.

19. Pérez Rodrigo C, Aranceta J, Salvador G, et al. Food frequency questionnaires. Nutr Hosp 2015;31(Suppl 3):49–56.

20. Paillard F, Flageul O, Mahé G, et al. Validation and reproducibility of a short food frequency questionnaire for cardiovascular prevention. Arch Cardiovasc Dis 2021;114(8–9):570–6.

21. White JV, Guenter P, Jensen G, et al. Consensus statement: Academy of Nutrition and Dietetics and American Society for Parenteral and Enteral Nutrition: characteristics recommended for the identification and documentation of adult malnutrition (undernutrition). JPEN J Parenter Enteral Nutr 2012;36(3):275–83.

22. Gillis C, Wischmeyer PE. Pre-operative nutrition and the elective surgical patient: why, how and what? Anaesthesia 2019;74(Suppl 1):27–35.

23. Wischmeyer PE, Carli F, Evans DC, et al. American Society for Enhanced Recovery and Perioperative Quality Initiative Joint Consensus Statement on Nutrition Screening and Therapy Within a Surgical Enhanced Recovery Pathway. Anesth Analg 2018;126(6):1883–95.

24. Esper DH. Utilization of nutrition-focused physical assessment in identifying micronutrient deficiencies. Nutr Clin Pract 2015;30(2):194–202.

25. Capone K, Sentongo T. The ABCs of Nutrient Deficiencies and Toxicities. Pediatr Ann 2019;48(11):e434–40.

26. DiBaise M, Tarleton SM. Hair, Nails, and Skin: Differentiating Cutaneous Manifestations of Micronutrient Deficiency. Nutr Clin Pract 2019;34(4):490–503.
27. André HP, Sperandio N, Siqueira RL, et al. Food and nutrition insecurity indicators associated with iron deficiency anemia in Brazilian children: a systematic review. Cien Saude Colet 2018;23(4):1159–67. Indicadores de insegurança alimentar e nutricional associados à anemia ferropriva em crianças brasileiras: uma revisão sistemática.
28. Bechthold A, Boeing H, Schwedhelm C, et al. Food groups and risk of coronary heart disease, stroke and heart failure: A systematic review and dose-response meta-analysis of prospective studies. Crit Rev Food Sci Nutr 2019;59(7):1071–90.
29. Schulze MB, Martínez-González MA, Fung TT, et al. Food based dietary patterns and chronic disease prevention. Bmj 2018;361:k2396.
30. Uusitupa M, Khan TA, Viguiliouk E, et al. Prevention of Type 2 Diabetes by Lifestyle Changes: A Systematic Review and Meta-Analysis. Nutrients 2019;11(11). https://doi.org/10.3390/nu11112611.
31. Rees K, Takeda A, Martin N, et al. Mediterranean-style diet for the primary and secondary prevention of cardiovascular disease. Cochrane Database Syst Rev 2019;3(3):Cd009825.
32. Ge L, Sadeghirad B, Ball GDC, et al. Comparison of dietary macronutrient patterns of 14 popular named dietary programmes for weight and cardiovascular risk factor reduction in adults: systematic review and network meta-analysis of randomised trials. Bmj 2020;369:m696.
33. Marincic PZ, Salazar MV, Hardin A, et al. Diabetes Self-Management Education and Medical Nutrition Therapy: A Multisite Study Documenting the Efficacy of Registered Dietitian Nutritionist Interventions in the Management of Glycemic Control and Diabetic Dyslipidemia through Retrospective Chart Review. J Acad Nutr Diet 2019;119(3):449–63.
34. Rozga M, Burrowes JD, Byham-Gray LD, et al. Effects of Sodium-Specific Medical Nutrition Therapy from a Registered Dietitian Nutritionist in Individuals with Chronic Kidney Disease: An Evidence Analysis Center Systematic Review and Meta-Analysis. J Acad Nutr Diet 2022;122(2):445–60.e19.

Awkward Topics
Discussing Weight with Your Patients

Mindy Haar, PhD, RDN, CDN, FAND[a],*, Rachel Hercman, LCSW[b]

KEYWORDS

- Obesity • Overweight • Weight management • Weight stigma • Nutrition Counseling
- Talking about weight

KEY POINTS

- Obesity rates are increasing with mounting evidence of links to chronic disease.
- Many health professionals are biased toward individuals with obesity and overweight thus creating weight stigma. This may prevent individuals from accessing the health-care system and health providers from effectively communicating about weight.
- Creating a sensitive, caring environment with attention to language and nonverbal communication can help change patient perception of bias and judgment.
- Individualized approaches to behavior and lifestyle change should be used.

BACKGROUND

The rates of individuals with obesity and overweight are increasing. Recent statistics from National Health and Nutrition Examination Survey indicate a national obesity rate of 42% (up from 30.5% in 1999–2000) and severe obesity at 9.2% (up from 4.7% 1999–2000).[1] Parallel with this increase in average weight is the incidence of type 2 diabetes mellitus. To date, 34.2 million people (10.5% of the US population) have type 2 diabetes, whereas 88 million adults (34.5% of the US population) have prediabetes.[2] In addition, obesity and overweight carry a higher risk for heart disease,[3] renal disease, and some types of cancer.[4] The relationship between adipose tissue and the immune system has been demonstrated with increased morbidity and mortality from coronavirus disease among those with obesity.[5]

The body mass index (BMI), a calculation of weight in kilograms divided by height in meters squared, is used as a screening tool.[6] It has limitations for diagnosing fatness and health but can be part of an assessment to evaluate health status and risks. Overweight is defined as having a BMI of 25, with obesity defined as more than 30, and

[a] Department of Interdisciplinary Health Sciences, Undergraduate Affairs, School of Health Professions, New York Institute of Technology, Riland 366, Old Westbury, NY 11568, USA;
[b] Psychotherapist in Private Practice, 27 West 96th, Street, New York, NY 10025, USA
* Corresponding author.
E-mail address: mhaar@nyit.edu

Physician Assist Clin 7 (2022) 589–598
https://doi.org/10.1016/j.cpha.2022.06.001
physicianassistant.theclinics.com

severe obesity, a BMI greater than 40. Although BMI is not a direct measure of body fat, it has a moderate correlation with more direct measures and a strong correlation with disease and metabolic outcomes. Waist circumference is another anthropometric measure that may help screen for risks associated with overweight and obesity as excess abdominal adipose tissue mass increases the risk of cardiovascular disease and type 2 Diabetes.[7] Men with a waist circumference greater than 40 inches and women with a waist circumference above 35 inches are at increased risk.

The relationship between weight and chronic and acute diseases obviates health-care practitioners to consider nutrition and lifestyle as an essential part of treatment.[8] However, this topic must be addressed with sensitivity to ensure the patient's comfort and increase the possibility of positive change.[9]

Society's attitudes toward weight may influence an individual's weight bias and judgment of others[10] and is referred to as weight stigma when this bias is toward those in larger bodies.[11] Research indicates a pervasiveness of weight bias both within American culture as well among health-care professionals.[12] When patients feel stigmatized, they may choose to avoid seeing a health-care professional, thereby exacerbating possible illness and chronic disease. Potential psychological effects include anxiety, depression, body image dissatisfaction, and disordered eating.[9] This may further snowball to losing motivation to exercise, increased stress, and possibly, further weight gain.

At the root of the existence of weight stigma is a belief that those with obesity or overweight lack willpower and willingness to do hard work[9]; the chronic diseases they experience are their own fault due to their laziness and lack of motivation.[13] A shift has begun, though, to recognition of myriad other factors affecting weight that include environmental exposures, genetics, and lack of access to optimal foods.[8] Thus, care must be taken by the health-care professional to examine their feelings about their own and others' body weight and approach conversations about weight with a nonjudgmental attitude.

To reduce stigma, some have proposed removing weight as a focus and instead use a "weight-inclusive" or "weight-neutral" approach.[9] This approach emphasizes reinforcing positive health behaviors regardless of changes in body weight.[14] In some instances, this has created a division with those advocating a "normative-weight" paradigm where weight loss can be a defined goal of improving health.[9]

Health at every size has emerged as a weight-neutral approach that promotes healthy daily practices, self-acceptance, and intuitive eating (IE) rather than restrictive diets resulting in weight loss.[13] IE focuses on guiding food intake in response to physiologic hunger and satiety cues rather than external, nonphysiological, cues such as food availability, emotions, smelling or seeing food, portion sizes, packaging, or social setting that encourage eating.[15] Mindful eating consists of paying attention to and experiencing food during consumption with the expectation that this awareness can lead to selection of healthier choices. Some research has indicated that those following this approach alone, which includes increased movement and exercise, can improve blood pressure and blood lipids and improve physical and psychological well-being.[13,16]

DISCUSSION
External Influences on Eating Behavior

There are individual differences in physiologic regulation of appetite and satiety, and metabolic rate that can be related to age, gender, physical activity, and comorbidities.[8] Eating behavior is also affected by external influences that include the following:

- Nutrition literacy: Nutrition literacy is the degree to which individuals can acquire, process, and synthesize basic nutrition information and services they need, enabling better nutrition choices.[17] Higher levels of nutrition literacy are related to higher quality and more healthful diets, which in turn are linked to lower diet-related chronic disease risk. Evaluating a patient's nutrition literacy can help the practitioner better tailor recommendations. Literacy can be subdivided as follows.[18]
  - Appreciating the importance of nutrition and knowledge of dietary guidelines to maintain wellness and prevent disease. This includes identifying nutrients and recognizing food groups.
  - Knowing how to get and evaluate nutrition information from sources such as nutrition labels and front of package claims.
  - Being able to apply nutrition information in making decisions on what to eat, how to budget and access food, and how to prepare food.

Although basic questions can be asked in this area, formal tools have been developed to measure nutrition literacy. The Rapid Eating Assessment for Patients is one such tool[19,20] that can be used in tandem with the Surveillance of Fruit and Vegetable Intake.[21] Newer tools such as Nutrition Literacy Assessment Instrument and Electronic Nutrition Literacy Assessment Tool have been validated and shown to predict adherence to healthful dietary patterns.[18,22]

- The food environment: The food industry seeks to manufacture foods that can override the body's ability to regulate calorie consumption and weight. Overconsumption can be related to foods made with specific combinations of sugar, salt, and fat that can have almost addictive qualities and extreme processing associated with hyperpalatability.[23,24] Ultraprocessed foods are responsible for most calories consumed in the United States.[25] Perception of normal portion sizes has been distorted as well as the message that it is acceptable to eat all day in all locations.[24]
- Economic price systems: Often energy-dense foods such as fast food and pasta are much lower priced than filling but nutrient-dense vegetables and fruits.[4,8] This makes making recommendations for an improved eating plan more challenging.
- Access and availability of healthier foods: Those who live in areas with a higher density of fast-food restaurants, fewer farmers' markets, or similar sources of fresh produce consume higher calorie diets.[8] Having adequate kitchen facilities affects the ability to prepare nutrient-dense meals as well as willingness and time to prepare meals.
- Social support: Eating patterns are influenced by those an individual encounters on a daily basis and can include family members and friends.[4,8] These individuals may be supportive of one's attempt to improve diet patterns and those living in the same household may be willing as a group to make changes. In other situations, this support may be lacking or efforts to make changes somewhat sabotaged. Technology has dramatically expanded the breadth of social connections a person can experience and this is particularly pertinent for issues of weight and diet: In one author's (R.H.) practice, there has been an increase in clients referencing social media communities as sources of information and misinformation as well as a sense of belonging and identification. Thus, speaking to a patient about weight and diet touches not only on their health but also on their confidence in what they know, who they know, and where they have come to feel comfortable socially.

Patient-Centered Approach

Thus, an individualized, patient-centered approach that considers the many variables contributing to weight should promote the following:[8]

1. *Examine and recognize biases that may affect the discussion of weight.* The UConn Rudd Center for Food Policy and Health has free training modules that promote a nonjudgmental attitude and elucidate the consequences of health biases.[26] They also provide a toolkit for health professionals for use in their practices.

   Bias may affect nonverbal communication as well.[27] Practitioners should maintain eye contact with the patient rather than at an electronic health record, written chart or table of normal weight BMI. When a patient in a larger body is sitting in your office, they presumably know they are overweight and may have received shaming messages from other providers. However, when there is a frame of warmth and caring about them not as an overweight person but as a person, there is a better chance for rapport and productive conversation.

2. *Check office space and equipment.* Be sure that chairs, gowns, blood pressure cuffs, and scales can accommodate diverse body sizes.[9]
3. *Pay attention to typical language.* To use *person-first* language, practitioners should describe an individual with a characteristic instead of the characteristic describing them as a person.[9,28] Thus, the conversation would include statements such as "There is an increased risk for diabetes for people with obesity" rather than "in obese people."[9]

   Rather than weight, prioritize health outcomes and behaviors and use empowering and supportive language without casting blame or shame.[29] Aside from how a practitioner refers to body weight, discussion of physical activity and eating habits may also include inadvertent stigma. Typical phrases used by health-care providers may communicate that people with obesity or overweight cannot resist temptation, lack discipline, cheat, and/or make excuses. The UConn Rudd Center for Food Policy & Health suggests the alternative phrases listed in **Box 1** to increase sensitivity:[29]

4. *Utilize motivational interviewing.* Motivational interviewing emphasizes a collaborative and supportive atmosphere between the health-care practitioner and the patient.[8] Instead of the practitioner dictating the plan, the practitioner evokes the patient's personal motives regarding changing a health-impacting behavior. Because this is in line with autonomy and patient choice, self-efficacy is enhanced, which is vital for changing and sustaining new changes.

Ask Questions such as[9]:

- What nutrition-related goals do you have?

Box 1 Communication Considerations	
Instead of saying…	**Try talking about…**
excuses	strategies to minimize triggers
discipline or self-control	ways to practice healthy habits as part of daily routines
cheat	situations that create challenges or difficulties
resist temptation	ways to cope with emotions that interfere with eating
do not overindulge	ways to feel satisfied and avoid feeling deprived
With permission from UConn Rudd Center for Food & Policy	

- What changes can you make?
- What are your anticipated challenges?
- What has worked for you in the past that may be revisited?

The UConn Rudd Center for Food Policy & Obesity provides detailed scripts for motivational interviewing during multiple patient visits.[30] Because patients may be in different stages of readiness to make changes, the conversation may be somewhat different: Patients may be thinking about making changes (precontemplation state), may be ambivalent about change (contemplation stage), or preparing to change and making small changes (preparation stage). Practitioners may first be seeing the patient when they are already in the preparation stage.

In the early precontemplation stage, it is important to validate the patient's autonomy by stating "It's your decision when you're ready to change your lifestyle," as well simply relaying your viewpoint of medical benefits of healthier eating by saying, "I note that your current eating patterns are increasing your risk for conditions such as type 2 diabetes and heart disease and making some changes in your lifestyle may result in substantial health improvements."[30] The practitioner can validate the patient's feelings of pressure from multiple sources and ambivalence about beginning to make changes.

During the contemplation stage, the practitioner can provide further validation of the patient's experience and autonomy.[30] Clarifying perceptions of the pros and cons of lifestyle change can be made with statements such as "What would be a positive result of making a change in eating patterns and what would be a negative result of making a change?" Further self-exploration could be encouraged with a request to think about the possibility to discuss by the next visit.

Because acknowledgment of the benefits of change and taking action begins in the preparation stage, the practitioner can further reinforce the decision.[30] Assistance can be given in prioritizing change opportunities by statements such as "In a review of your eating habits, a big benefit would come from reducing the amount of sugar in the multiple cups of coffee you drink each day. Do you agree?" In addition, a discussion of experience with making previous changes and what worked and what did not would be appropriate, as well as identifying obstacles and strategies for dealing with them.

5. *Emphasize the importance of small changes.* Weight loss and maintenance of just 3% to 5% of original weight has demonstrated clinically important health improvements.[8] These changes include reductions in triglycerides, blood glucose, and type 2 diabetes risk. When a greater percentage of weight is lost, at least 5% to 10%, reduction in cholesterol and blood pressure may result as well as a decreased need for medication to control cardiovascular disease and type 2 diabetes. Many find changing habits more manageable when viewed from the perspective of 1 day at a time and more reachable goals.

6. *Prioritize the need for long-term, sustainable lifestyle changes.* Those successful at maintaining their desired body weight do not view lifestyle changes as something taken on and then abandoned but rather lifelong adjustments in eating and activity.[8,31] Elucidate to patients that once weight is lost, the lower weight requires reduced energy; thus, returning to original energy intake will not maintain a new lower weight. It has been one author's (M.H.) experience with thousands of patients in 43 years of practice to have encountered zero individuals who maintained weight loss after a "fad diet" type regimen.

As intensive behavioral and lifestyle treatment of those with obesity or overweight is being used successfully in treatments and prevention of type 2 diabetes and other chronic diseases, it is increasingly being recognized as a mainstream approach and covered by insurance reimbursement.[32]

7. *Discuss mindfulness.* Strategies to increase awareness of the eating experience to maximize response to physiologic cues to eat and feel satiated include:[33]
   - Being aware of hunger level and of possible emotional triggers to eat
   - Noticing smell, taste, and texture of food
   - Sitting while eating
   - Avoiding doing other activities while eating
   - Eating more slowly (putting down utensils between bites can help)
   - Planning snacks and meals in advance

8. *Recognize that one size does not fit all.* Individuals embarking on behavior change may find different approaches that work for them, and some may use a combination of methods.[8] For some, focusing on IE and mindfulness may be sufficient, whereas others find the need for more structured approaches.
   - Specific food recommendations: The Dietary Guidelines for Americans, 2020-2025, Mediterranean Diet and Dietary Approach to Stop Hypertension all emphasize moving to more plant-based food patterns with more fruits, vegetables, nuts, legumes, whole grains with preference for fish and poultry over higher fat meat.[34] These approaches also recommend reduction of sugar and processed foods.
   - Commercial programs such as Weight Watchers emphasize point systems and portion control along with varying levels of live and virtual group feedback and engagement.[35]
   - Twelve-step fellowships: For some with obesity, their weight reflects compulsive eating and/or compulsive food behaviors.[36] Groups such as Overeaters Anonymous treat obesity from the perspective of a disease model.
   - Regular weighing: Although not all approaches promote regular weighing, some individuals find the feedback from knowing their weight on a monthly, weekly, or even daily basis beneficial.[8] For these people, this knowledge allows for healthful readjustment in food intake to reach or maintain a desirable weight. For others, this can be discouraging and possibly reflect or lead to disordered eating and/or eating disorders.
   - Tracking food and activity: Some individuals find tracking through journals or apps increases awareness and mindfulness of what they eat and daily movement.[8]

9. *Acknowledge environmental and social factors that may affect your recommendations and patient success.*[9] The practitioner should ensure that discussion of weight correlates with the patient's ability to make changes, their finances, their food environment, family support, and cultural preferences.

10. *Include discussion of exercise.* Current recommendations suggest engaging in moderate-intensity exercise 150 to 300 minutes or 75 to 150 minutes of more vigorous exercise each week with muscle strengthening activities done at least twice weekly.[37] The most recent government guidelines mention that duration of individual exercise bouts can be less than 10 minutes. Thus, for those who may not have a 30 to 60 minute period to exercise, including several "exercise snacks" throughout the day can help achieve physical fitness. Many find this beneficial to appetite control and mood.

11. *Explore resources for practitioner nutrition knowledge.* The American Association of Physician Assistants,[38] Physicians Committee for Responsible Medicine,[39] US Department of Health and Human Services,[40] the US Department of Agriculture (USDA),[41] all provide toolkits for health professionals who assist patients wishing

to improve their dietary patterns. Some include opportunities for continuing education credits.

In addition, practitioners can benefit from taking a nutrition course through an accredited institution or completing an Advanced Certificate for Healthcare Professionals.[42]

12. *Provide resources to patients to support health goals.* Resources should be made available through hard copies or electronic links. An array of excellent free handouts in multiple languages are available as part of practitioner toolkits listed above as well as from organizations such as the Academy of Nutrition and Dietetics,[43,44] Dietary Guidelines for Americans,[45] and UC Davis Health.[46] The USDA's nutrition.gov division provides handouts as well on My Plate and other topics.[47,48]

13. *Include Registered Dietitian-Nutritionists (RDNs) as part of the intervention team.* Comprehensive and multiple sessions are often needed with an expert nutrition professional to support a patient in successfully changing their eating habits.[8,49] Some medical practices can use RDNs on staff full-time or part-time. When this is not possible, the Academy of Nutrition and Dietetics hosts a list of RDNs in practice by zip code who provide both in-office and telehealth availability to whom referrals can be made.[50]

14. *Facilitate ongoing support even when long-term goals are reached.* Patients may be dealing with gradual weight regain due to increased appetite and/or inaccurate perception of increasing portion sizes.[25] Emphasizing improvement of blood pressure and glycemic control can spur motivation to continue with lifestyle changes as well as experience the health-care practitioners' support and collaboration on maintaining goals.

SUMMARY

Obesity rates are increasing in the United States while evidence continues to support its relationship to chronic disease. Health-care professionals often approach the discussion of weight with judgment, further alienating patients from getting the care they need. Many factors affect patient weight and include physiologic, psychological, environmental, economic influences as well as nutrition literacy. Providers may optimize chances for patient lifestyle change when they examine their own biases, moderate their language, attend to their nonverbal communication, use motivational interviewing, emphasize the impact of small but sustainable changes, consider individualized approaches, and include nutrition professionals as part of the health-care team.

CLINICS CARE POINTS

- As weight stigma may lead to avoidance of medical care for those in need, providers should examine potential bias in their patient communications.

- Allow patients to set their own goals and collaborate with them to find nutrition approaches that work for them.

- Weight reduction and maintenance of just 3% to 5% of original weight may reduce triglycerides, blood glucose, and type 2 diabetes risk while at least 5% to 10% is associated with a reduction in cholesterol and blood pressure.

- Nutrition professionals can provide the necessary time and support to patients seeking lifestyle changes when included as part of the medical team.

DISCLOSURE

The authors have nothing to disclose.

REFERENCES

1. Hales DM, Carroll MD, Fryar C, et al. Prevalence of obesity and severe obesity among adults: United States, 2017-2018. Updated February 2020. Available at: https://www.cdc.gov/nchs/data/databriefs/db360-h.pdf. Accessed January 9, 2022.
2. Centers for Disease Control and Prevention. National Diabetes Statistics Report. Available at: https://www.cdc.gov/diabetes/data/statistics-report/index.html. Accessed January 9, 2022.
3. Centers for Disease Control and Prevention. Prevent Heart Disease. 2022. Available at: https://www.cdc.gov/heartdisease/prevention.htm. Accessed January 17, 2022.
4. Office of Disease Prevention and Health Promotion. Healthy People 2020 Topics and Objectives: Nutrition and Weight Status. 2021. Available at: https://www.healthypeople.gov/2020/topics-objectives/topic/nutrition-and-weight-status. Accessed January 9, 2022.
5. Centers for Disease Control and Prevention. Division of Nutrition PAaO. Obesity, Race/Ethnicity, and COVID-19. 2022. Available at: https://www.cdc.gov/obesity/data/obesity-and-covid-19.html. Accessed January 9, 2022.
6. Center for Disease Control and Prevention. Healthy weight, nutrition and physical activity: About adult BMI. Available at: https://www.cdc.gov/healthyweight/assessing/bmi/adult_bmi/. Accessed January 17, 2022.
7. Ross R, Neeland IJ, Yamashita S, et al. Waist circumference as a vital sign in clinical practice: a Consensus Statement from the IAS and ICCR Working Group on Visceral Obesity. Nat Rev Endocrinol 2020;16(3):177–89.
8. Raynor HA, Champagne CM. Position of the Academy of Nutrition and Dietetics: Interventions for Treatment of Overweight and Obesity in Adults. J Acad Nutr Diet 2016;119(1):129–47.
9. Howes EM, Harden SM, Cox HK, et al. Communicating about weight in dietetics practice: Recommendations for reducation of weight bias and stigma. J Acad Nutr Diet 2021;121(9):1669–73.
10. Anderson J, Bresnahan M. Communicating stigma about body size. Health Commun 2013;28(6):603–15.
11. Puhl RM, Himmelstein MS, Pearl RL. Weight stigma as a psychosocial contributor to obesity. Am Psychol 2020;75(2):274–89.
12. Lawrence BJ, Kerr D, Pollard CM, et al. Weight bias among health care professionals: A systematic review and meta-analysis. Obesity 2021;29(11):1802–12.
13. Rauchwerk A, Vipperman-Cohen A, Padmanabhan S, et al. The case for a health at every size approach for chronic disease risk reduction in women of color. J Nutr Educ Behav 2020;52(11):1066–72.
14. Tylka TL, Annunziato RA, Burgard D, et al. The weight-inclusive versus weight-normative approach to health: evaluating the evidence for prioritizing well-being over weight loss. J Obes 2014;2014:983495.
15. Grider HS, Douglas SM, Raynor HA. The influence of mindful eating and/or intuitive eating approaches on dietary intake: A systematic review. J Acad Nutr Diet 2021;121(4):709–727 e1.
16. Huebner GE, McGuirt JT, Perrin MT, et al. Nondiet weight-neutral curricula limited in curent accredited US dietetic programs. J Nutr Educ Behav 2021;53(6):517–23.

17. Marchello NJ, Daley CM, Sullivan DK, et al. Nutrition literacy tailored interventions may improve diet behaviors in outpatient nutrition clinics. J Nutr Educ Behav 2021;53(12):1048–54.
18. Franklin J, Holman C, Tam R, et al. Validation of the e-NutLit, an electronic tool to assess nutrition literacy. J Nutr Educ Behav 2020;52(6):607–14.
19. Gans KM, Risica PM, Wylie-Rosett J, et al. Development and evaluation of the nutrition component of the Rapid Eating and Activity Assessment for Patients (REAP): a new tool for primary care providers. J Nutr Educ Behav 2006;38(5):286–92.
20. Gans KM. Rapid eating assessment for patients (REAP). Available at: https://www.brown.edu/academics/public-health/chphe/sites/public-health-cher/files/Reap7.pdf. Accessed January 23, 2022.
21. Centers for Disease Control and Prevention. Data user's guide to the BRFSS Fruit and Vegetable Module. Available at: https://www.cdc.gov/nutrition/data-statistics/data-users-guide.html. Accessed January 23, 2022.
22. Taylor MK, Sullivan DK, Ellerbeck EF, et al. Nutrition literacy predicts adherence to healthy/unhealthy diet patterns in adults with a nutrition-related chronic condition. Public Health Nutr 2019;22(12):2157–69.
23. Roberto CA, Swinburn B, Hawkes C, et al. Patchy progress on obesity prevention: emerging examples, entrenched barriers, and new thinking. Lancet 2015; 385(9985):2400–9.
24. Brownell KD. Thinking forward: the quicksand of appeasing the food industry. Plos Med 2012;9(7). https://doi.org/10.1371/journal.pmed.1001254. e1001254-e1001254.
25. Hall KD, Kahan S. Maintenance of lost weight and long-term management of obesity. Med Clin North Am 2018;102(1):183–97.
26. Rudd Center for Food Policy & Health UConn. Healthcare Providers/Resources/Training Modules. Available at: https://uconnruddcenter.org/research/weight-bias-stigma/healthcare-providers/. Accessed January 19, 2022.
27. Puhl RM, Phelan SM, Nadglowski J, et al. Overcoming weight bias in the management of patients With diabetes and obesity. Clin Diabetes 2016;34(1):44–50.
28. Fruh SM, Graves RJ, Hauff C, et al. Weight bias and stigma: Impact on health. Nurs Clin North Am 2021;56(4):479–93.
29. UConn Rudd Center for Food Policy & Health. Reducing stigma talking to patients. Available at: https://uconnruddcenter.org/wp-content/uploads/sites/2909/2020/11/Reducing-Stigma-Talking-to-Patients.pdf. Accessed January 19, 2022.
30. UConn Rudd Center for Food Policy & Health. Motivational interviewing: Example scripts. Available at: https://uconnruddcenter.org/wp-content/uploads/sites/2909/2020/07/Motivational-Interviewing-Example-Scrip. Accessed January 19, 2022.
31. Wing RR, Phelan SM. Long-term weight loss maintenance. Americal J Clin Nutr 2005;82(1):222S–5S.
32. Williamson DA. Fifty years of behavioral/lifestyle interventions for overweight and obesity: Where have we been and where are we going? Obesity (Silver Spring) 2017;25(11):1867–75.
33. Warren JM, Smith N, Ashwell M. A structured literature review on the role of mindfulness, mindful eating and intuitive eating in changing eating behaviours: effectiveness and associated potential mechanisms. Nutr Res Rev 2017;30(2):272–83.
34. Lavie CJ, Laddu D, Arena R, et al. Healthy weight and obesity prevention: JACC health promotion series. J Am Coll Cardiol 2018;72(13):1506–31.
35. Thomas JG, Raynor HA, Bond DS, et al. Weight loss in Weight Watchers online with and without an activity tracking device compared to control: A randomized trial. Obesity (Silver Spring) 2017;25(6):1014–21.

36. Bray B, Rodriguez-Martin BC, Wiss DA, et al. Overeaters anonymous: An overlooked intervention for binge eating disorder. Int J Environ Res Public Health 2021;18(14). https://doi.org/10.3390/ijerph18147303.

37. US Department of Health and Human Services. Physican Activity Guidelines for American. 2nd edition. Available at: https://health.gov/sites/default/files/2019-09/Physical_Activity_Guidelines_2nd_edition.pdf. Accessed January 23, 2022.

38. American Association of Physician Assistants. Nutrition Toolkit. Available at: https://www.aapa.org/cme-central/national-health-priorities/nutrition-toolkit/#tabs-3-patient-education-resources. Accessed January 23, 2022.

39. Physicians Committee for Responsible Medicine. Nutrition for clinicians. Available at: https://www.pcrm.org/good-nutrition/nutrition-for-clinicians. Accessed January 23, 2022.

40. US Department of Health and Human Services. Office of Disease Prevention and Health Promotion. Toolkit for health professionals. Available at: https://health.gov/our-work/nutrition-physical-activity/dietary-guidelines/current-dietary-guidelines/toolkit-professionals. Accessed January 23, 2021.

41. US Department of Agriculture Food and Nutrition Information Center. Information for Health Professionals. Available at: https://www.nal.usda.gov/legacy/fnic/information-health-professionals. Accessed January 23, 2022.

42. New York Institute of Technology. Nutrition for Healthcare Providers, Advanced Certificate. Available at: https://www.nyit.edu/degrees/nutrition_for_healthcare_providers_ac. Accessed February 20, 2022.

43. Academy of Nutrition and Dietetics. Food and nutrition handouts in multiple languages. Available at: https://www.eatrightpro.org/about-us/what-is-an-rdn-and-dtr/work-with-an-rdn-or-dtr/food-and-nutrition-handouts-in-multiple-languages. Accessed January 23, 2022.

44. Academy of Nutrition and Dietetics. Eat right nutrition tips and handouts. Available at: https://www.eatrightpro.org/practice/career-development/marketing-center/eat-right-nutrition-tips-and-handouts.

45. Dietary Guidelines for Americans. Consumer resources. Available at: https://www.dietaryguidelines.gov/resources/consumer-resources. Accessed January 23, 2022.

46. Davis Health/Food and Nutrition Services UC. Nutrition education materials. Available at: https://health.ucdavis.edu/food-nutrition/nutritionservices/nutritioneducationmaterials.html. Accessed January 23, 2022.

47. US Department of Agriculture Food and Nutrition. gov. Printable materials and handouts. Available at: https://www.nutrition.gov/topics/basic-nutrition/printable-materials-and-handouts. Accessed January 23, 2022.

48. US Department of Agriculture Food. My Plate. Available at: https://www.myplate.gov/. Accessed January 30 ,2022.

49. Cheng FW, Garay JL, Handu D. Weight management Interventions for adults with overweight or obesity: An evidence analysis center scoping review. J Acad Nutr Diet 2021;121(9):1855–65.

50. Academy of Nutrition and Dietetics. Find a nutrition expert. Available at: https://www.eatright.org/find-a-nutrition-expert. Accessed January 22, 2022.

Introduction to the Nutrients and Their Association with Common Gastrointestinal Disorders

Corri Wolf, PhD, PA-C, RDN[a],*, Richard N. Steller, MD[b]

KEYWORDS

- Carbohydrate • Protein • Fat • Celiac disease • Gluten • Irritable bowel syndrome
- FODMAP • Gastroparesis

KEY POINTS

- A well-balanced diet includes six classes of nutrients: protein, carbohydrates, fat, vitamins, minerals, and water. Although most foods are a blend of energy-yielding nutrients (protein, carbohydrate, and fat), a food is usually classified by its predominant nutrient.
- Gluten is a complex of water-insoluble proteins found in the complex carbohydrates wheat, rye, barley, and hybrids of these grains; avoiding these grains is the only acceptable treatment for celiac disease.
- Dietary therapies for irritable bowel syndrome are gaining increasing attention; to date, the largest body of literature pertains to the low fermentable oligosaccharides, disaccharides, monosaccharides, and polyols (FODMAP) diet.
- Dietary protein is required as a source of amino acids. Protein restriction should not be prescribed in patients with impaired hepatic function as it increases protein catabolism and sarcopenia.
- Diet is the first line of treatment for gastroparesis and recent studies have focused on meal composition and specific trigger foods enabling practitioners to provide more evidence-based advice beyond simply recommending a low-fat diet.

INTRODUCTION

Poor nutrition has been associated with various diseases and most adults do not eat a healthy, well-balanced diet.[1] As indicated in the Dietary Guidelines for Americans 2020 to 2025, following a healthy dietary pattern can help achieve and maintain good health and reduce the risk of chronic diseases throughout the lifespan.[2] A well-balanced diet includes six classes of nutrients: protein, carbohydrate, fat,

[a] Department of Physician Assistant Studies, School of Health Professions, New York Institute of Technology, Old Westbury, NY 11568, USA; [b] Gastroenterology, Medical Director, Catholic Health Physician Partners at Merrick, 131 Merrick Road, Merrick, NY 11566, USA
* Corresponding author.
E-mail address: cwolf01@nyit.edu

Physician Assist Clin 7 (2022) 599–613
https://doi.org/10.1016/j.cpha.2022.05.004
2405-7991/22/© 2022 Elsevier Inc. All rights reserved.

vitamins, minerals, and water. Nutrients have at least one of three primary functions: they provide energy, contribute to body structure, and regulate chemical processes in the body.[3] The three macronutrients, namely protein, carbohydrate, and fat, are energy-yielding and produce energy during metabolism to fuel metabolic and physical activities (**Table 1**). Vitamins, minerals, and water do not supply energy. Although it provides calories, alcohol offers no advantage as a fuel and is not a nutrient.[4]

Table 1 Sources of energy	
Source	**Kilocalories (kcal)**
Protein	4 kcal/gram
Carbohydrate	4 kcal/gram
Alcohol	7 kcal/gram
Fat	9 kcal/gram

Kilocalories (kcal)—measurement of the amount of energy that can be released by the macronutrients and alcohol.

Carbohydrates and fats are the primary fuel sources and can be utilized interchangeably although the body can only store unlimited amounts of fat, not carbohydrate. Furthermore, many metabolic processes favor one source over another. For instance, the brain functions almost exclusively on glucose under normal circumstances, and membranes are composed of specific lipids. Proteins are required for tissue maintenance, replacement, function, and growth. However, if the body lacks sufficient calories from dietary sources or tissue stores, protein may be used for energy .[4,5] Glucose from simple and complex carbohydrates is stored as glycogen in the liver and muscle when not needed for energy.[4]

Although most foods are a blend of energy-yielding nutrients, a food is usually classified by its predominant nutrient. For example, bread is classified as carbohydrate, egg as protein, and olive oil as fat. An additional way of classifying nutrients is as essential or nonessential. Essential nutrients cannot be synthesized by the human body or not synthesized in sufficient amounts for normal functioning. As a result, essential nutrients must be obtained from food. Conversely, nonessential nutrients can be synthesized in the body in sufficient quantities for normal functioning. However, these nutrients are also usually obtained from food.[6] Acceptable macronutrient distribution ranges (AMDRs), the percentage of calories from each macronutrient in regard to the overall daily intake, have been established for protein, carbohydrate, and fat to provide adequate nutrients and energy for healthy individuals and reduce the risk of chronic disease (**Table 2**).[5]

Table 2 Acceptable macronutrient distribution ranges	
Macronutrient	**Range (Percent of Energy)**
Protein	10–35
Carbohydrate	45–65
Fat	20–35

Considerations: Energy Density Versus Nutrient Density

Energy density is the amount of energy or calories in a specific amount of food per serving. Conversely, nutrient density is a measure of the nutrients a food provides relative to the energy it provides. The more nutrients and fewer calories, the higher the nutrient density. It is important to note that foods can also be both energy and nutrient dense.[7]

- Sugar is energy-dense but provides no vitamins or minerals.
- Broccoli isnutrient-dense but provides few calories.
- Avocado is both energy andnutrient-dense.

DISCUSSION: MACRONUTRIENTS
Carbohydrate

Simple carbohydrates
Carbohydrates are traditionally classified as simple or complex based on the number of sugar molecules in their chemical structures. Simple carbohydrates are further classifieds as monosaccharides or disaccharides (**Table 3**). Disaccharides are two monosaccharides linked together.[8]

Sugar alcohols can occur naturally or can be chemically synthesized derivatives of monosaccharides and disaccharides. Examples of sugar alcohols are sorbitol and xylitol. These substances are also called polyols and are used to sweeten foods. They are incompletely digested and absorbed; as a result, they are less caloric.[8]

Table 3 Simple carbohydrates	
Monosaccharides	
Glucose	Primary fuel for humans; brain dependent on it during normal conditions
Fructose	Found in fruits, honey, and sugarcane; used to make high fructose corn syrup to sweeten foods and beverages
Galactose	Primarily found in milk
Disaccharides	
Sucrose (Glucose + Fructose)	Table sugar; many fruits and vegetables; high concentration in sugar beets and sugarcane
Lactose (Glucose + Galactose)	Found in dairy products—milk, yogurt, cheese
Maltose (Glucose + Glucose)	Breakdown product of plant starches; rarely found in foods

Complex carbohydrates
Complex carbohydrates are polysaccharides and are composed of long chains of monosaccharides. The two main groups of polysaccharides are starches and fibers. Starches that predominate in the human diet are amylose and amylopectin and are primarily found in grains, grain products, root vegetables, and legumes. A small percentage of starch that is consumed is resistant to digestion. These resistant starches promote the growth of colonic bacteria, which break down these starches to short-chain fatty acids, providing nutrition to the colonic cells.[9,10]

Fiber is generally considered "roughage" that is indigestible; however, bacteria in the colon can break down these molecules. Most often, fiber is categorized by its solubility (soluble vs insoluble) and its physiologic effect (**Table 4**). In addition to its beneficial physiologic effects, such as lowering cholesterol, and improving blood sugar and bowel pattern, dietary fiber also improves the growth and activity of beneficial intestinal bacteria improving host health. Recent dietary fiber definitions have included various nondigestible carbohydrates in addition to nonstarch polysaccharides such as resistant starch, resistant maltodextrins, fructo-oligosaccharides, galacto-oligosaccharides, modified celluloses, and synthesized carbohydrate polymers.[10] Despite its known health benefits, the majority of Americans do not meet the recommended dietary guidelines for fiber, 14 g/1000 kcal, which is roughly 20 to 35 g/d depending on caloric needs.[2]

Table 4 Sources and physiologic properties of fiber[2,10]	
Soluble fiber: attracts water and turns to gel during digestion	Oat bran, barley, nuts, seeds, beans, lentils, peas, and some fruits and vegetables; psyllium (common fiber supplement)
Insoluble fiber: adds bulk to the stool	Wheat bran, vegetables, and whole grains

Clinical Relevance: Gastrointestinal Disorders Associated with Carbohydrate Metabolism

Celiac disease

Celiac Disease (CD) is a chronic small intestinal immune-mediated disorder precipitated by exposure to dietary gluten in genetically predisposed individuals.[11] Gluten is the complex of water-insoluble proteins found in wheat, rye, barley, and hybrids of these grains, such as triticale and kamut (**Table 5**). Medical nutrition therapy and avoiding these grains are the only acceptable treatment for celiac disease.[11,12]

Controversies: Oats

The North American Society for the Study of Celiac Disease (NASSCD) stated that most people with celiac disease could safely consume oats uncontaminated by wheat, barley, and rye. Furthermore, they acknowledged that oats add diversity and offer many nutritional benefits to the gluten-free diet.[13]

Alcohol and Celiac Disease

Most hard liquor, distilled liquors, and hard ciders are gluten-free. Even if these products are made from gluten-containing grains, they do not contain gluten peptides as they are too large to carry over in the distillation process. Beers, ales, lagers, and malt beverages made from gluten-containing grains are not distilled and therefore are not gluten-free. Wine is generally gluten-free, except those varieties with added

Table 5 Sources of gluten	
Wheat	Bread, baked goods, soups, pasta, cereals, sauces, salad dressing, roux _Varieties and derivatives of wheat_: wheatberries, durum, emmer, semolina, spelt, farina, farro, graham, kamut, khorasan wheat, einkorn wheat
Barley	Malt (malted barley flour, malted milk, and milkshakes, malt extract, malt syrup, malt flavoring, malt vinegar), food coloring, soups, beer, Brewer's yeast
Rye	Rye bread, rye beer, cereals
Triticale	Bread, pasta, cereals

Data From Celiac Disease Foundation: https://celiac.org/gluten-free-living/what-is-gluten/.

color or flavoring, for example, dessert wines. However, wines made from barley malt, such as, bottled wine coolers, contain gluten.[12]

Patient Education

The United States Food and Drug Administration (FDA) defined the term "gluten-free," and for a food or product to make that claim, it must contain less than 20 ppm of gluten.[14] Gluten is ubiquitous in the diet and often not readily identified on food labels. Furthermore, a gluten-free diet and use of gluten-free products were historically low in B vitamins, calcium, Vitamin D, iron, zinc, magnesium, and fiber, and few gluten-free products were enriched or fortified, adding to the risk of nutrient deficiencies.[12] However, there are now several nutrient-dense grains, seeds, legumes, and nut flours that offer increased variety, improved palatability, and add higher nutritional quality to the gluten-free diet. Therefore, patients must be educated by an experienced Registered Dietitian Nutritionist (RDN) on nutrient-dense foods that are gluten-free, label reading, and hidden sources of gluten (**Table 6**).

Table 6 Gluten-free foods	
Naturally gluten-free food groups	Fruits, vegetables, meat and poultry, fish and seafood, dairy, beans, legumes, and nuts
Naturally gluten-free grains	Amaranth, buckwheat cornmeal, hominy, millet, quinoa, rice, sorghum, teff

Data from Celiac Disease Foundation: https://celiac.org/gluten-free-living/what-is-gluten/.

Irritable bowel syndrome

Irritable bowel syndrome (IBS) is the most prevalent functional gastrointestinal disorder, and current estimates indicate it affects approximately 11% of adults globally.[15] Due to its prevalence, IBS poses a significant burden on the health care system. As patients experience abdominal pain and altered bowel habits in the absence of organic causes, dietary therapies for IBS are of increasing interest. To date, the largest body of literature pertains to the low fermentable oligosaccharides, disaccharides, monosaccharides, and polyols (FODMAP) diet, and results suggest a possible benefit for overall IBS symptoms in approximately half of those who suffer.[16] FODMAPs are fermentable short-chain carbohydrates found in everyday foods (**Table 7**).[17]

Table 7 FODMAPs[17]	
Fermentable	Short-Chain Carbohydrate Subtypes and Examples of Sources
Oligosaccharides	Fructans: wheat, onions, garlic, inulin, chicory root, pistachios, cashews, teas—chamomile/chai Galacto-oligosaccharides: beans, lentils, green peas, soybeans/milk
Disaccharides	Lactose: milk, yogurt, ice cream, cottage cheese, ricotta cheese
Monosaccharides	Fructose (in excess of glucose): high fructose corn syrup, honey, apples, pears, watermelon, mango, asparagus, artichoke, rum
And	
Polyols	Mannitol: cauliflower, mushrooms Sorbitol: blackberries, avocado, prunes Xylitol, maltitol, isomalt: candy, gum, mints sweetened with sugar-alcohols Medications: cough syrups, liquid nonsteroidals, and any suspensions, elixirs, etc.

Monosaccharides

Most of carbohydrate digestion and absorption occurs in the small intestine, and all carbohydrates must be broken down into monosaccharides for absorption. A sodium-dependent transporter moves the monosaccharides glucose and galactose into the enterocyte. Fructose is primarily absorbed through GLUT-5 transporter-mediated facilitative diffusion, and its absorptive capacity is carrier limited.[18] Glucose promotes intestinal fructose absorption in the small intestine, but excessive dietary intake of fructose can easily overwhelm the absorptive capacity leading to fructose malabsorption.[19] Research has demonstrated that the fructose:glucose ratio of 1:1 is ideal for absorption of fructose; higher proportions of fructose are malabsorbed.[20] The unabsorbed fructose creates an osmotic load that is rapidly driven into the colon where anaerobic flora ferments it producing gas, bloating, and diarrhea. Approximately half the US population cannot absorb greater than 25 g of fructose, yet the fructose content of many diets regularly exceeds 50 g, which 100% of humans cannot absorb.[19] High dietary fructose is often due to the ingestion of sweetened beverages, most often with high fructose corn syrup, manufactured from corn starch and used as an inexpensive way to sweeten products.

Disaccharides

Lactose is a disaccharide hydrolyzed to the monosaccharides glucose and galactose by intestinal lactase, located on the microvillus membrane of the intestinal absorptive cells. The sodium-dependent glucose carrier then facilitates the uptake of glucose and galactose. When lactose is not hydrolyzed, it passes from the small bowel to the colon, where it is transformed into short-chain fatty acids and hydrogen gas by the intestinal bacteria. If large amounts of lactose are malabsorbed, lactose and its fermentation products cause symptoms of intolerance: bloating, gas, and diarrhea.[21] Lactase persistence is genetically determined, and approximately two-thirds of the world's population undergoes a genetically programmed decrease (primary lactose intolerance).[22] Additionally, those with lactase persistence can experience a health issue that decreases lactase activity, such as a gastrointestinal infection, celiac disease, Crohn's disease, or bowel surgery (secondary lactose intolerance).

An individual's threshold for dietary lactose tolerance is variable and dependent on several factors, including the dose consumed, residual lactase present, ingestion with other dietary components, gut transit time, and composition of the individual's enteric microbiome.[21] Furthermore, most people with lactase nonpersistence can tolerate

Table 8 High-lactose foods	
Food	**Serving**
The following foods contain approximately 5 to 8 g of lactose:	
Milk (whole, reduced fat, fat-free, buttermilk, goat's milk)	1/2 cup
Evaporated milk	1/4 cup
Cheese spread and soft cheeses	2 oz.
Cottage cheese	3/4 cup
Ricotta cheese	3/4 cup
Yogurt, plain	1/2 cup
Ice cream	3/4 cup
Nonfat dry milk powder	2 Tbsp

Cleveland Clinic: https://my.clevelandclinic.org/health/diseases/7317-lactose-intolerance.

Table 9
Low-lactose foods

Food	Serving
The following foods contain approximately 0 to 2 g of lactose:	
Condensed milk	1/2 cup
Half and half	1/2 cup
Sour cream	2 tbsp
Milk, treated with lactase enzyme	1/2 cup
Sherbet	1/2 cup
Aged cheese (blue, brick, cheddar, Colby, Swiss, Parmesan)	1–2 oz.
Processed cheese	1 oz.

Cleveland Clinic: https://my.clevelandclinic.org/health/diseases/7317-lactose-intolerance.

small amounts of lactose, 12 to 15 g, especially when combined with other foods or spread throughout the day (**Tables 8** and **9**).[23]

Patient Education

Milk and dairy are the primary sources of dietary calcium, an essential nutrient. However, calcium can also be found in nondairy sources (**Table 10**).

Table 10
Non-dairy sources of calcium

Food	Serving	Calcium
Sardines	3 oz.	325 mg
Spinach (cooked)	1 cup	240 mg
Broccoli (cooked)	1 cup	180 mg
Calcium-fortified orange juice	8 oz.	350 mg
Calcium-fortified soy or almond milk	8 oz.	300 mg
Dried beans (cooked)	1 1/2 cup	150 mg
Tofu	1/2 cup	250 mg

Cleveland Clinic: https://my.clevelandclinic.org/health/diseases/7317-lactose-intolerance.

Patients should not avoid or restrict dairy. They can enjoy dairy and ensure adequate calcium intake using the lactase enzyme, available without prescription in liquid, tablet, or chewable form. Patients should take the enzyme with lactose-containing foods. However, if eating out, they should take it even if their meal does not contain obvious dairy as it is often consumed without one realizing it.

Oligosaccharides and Polyols

As previously mentioned, humans lack the enzymes to digest and absorb these carbohydrates, and eating foods that contain them can cause bloating, gas, and diarrhea. To categorize a food as a high or low FODMAP, a cutoff value per serving has been established for all FODMAPs, including fructo-oligosaccharides (fructans) and galacto-oligosaccharides. Many fruits, vegetables, grains, nuts, and seeds exceed this established level. Similarly, a cutoff value has been established for polyols that are naturally found in the diet or manufactured.[24]

Low FODMAP Diet Implementation[17]

Three Phases:

1. Elimination Phase:

   Restrict all high FODMAP foods from the diet for 2 to 6 weeks.

2. Reintroduction Phase:

   Reintroduce small amounts of one food; gradually increase the dose over 2 to 3 days if the food is tolerated.
   If symptoms develop, discontinue that food for a 3 to 4 day washout period.
   When symptom-free, the next FODMAP challenge begins.
   The process typically lasts 6 to 8 weeks.

3. Maintenance Phase:

   Long-term adherence to a personalized modified diet is the goal.

Controversies: Long-Term Risks and Unanswered Questions

Limited data are available regarding the prolonged use of the FODMAP diet. This underscores the need to restrict the elimination phase to 6 weeks and advance the diet to the maintenance phase liberalizing it as much as individually possible. Areas of concern include the diet's effect on the microbiome and potentially being low in fiber. However, a recent study demonstrated no change in Bifidobacteria after 12 months on a personalized FODMAP diet.[25]

PROTEIN

Dietary protein is required as a source of amino acids. There are 20 amino acids, of which 9 are essential. The nonessential amino acids are considered dispensable and can be excluded from a diet as the body can synthesize them using only the essential amino acids.[6] Dietary protein requirements are weight-adjusted. The requirement for dietary protein correlates with growth rate, thus is the highest in infancy and the lowest in adults, 0.8 g/kg/d[9] This recommendation is based on nitrogen balance in healthy individuals.

Clinical Relevance: Gastrointestinal Disorders Associated with Protein Metabolism

Cirrhosis and hepatic encephalopathy

Protein is the only macronutrient that contains nitrogen. When catabolized to produce energy, nitrogenous waste is produced and is metabolized to urea for excretion. Nitrogenous intermediates, such as ammonia, are toxic when accumulated; this can become problematic when hepatic or renal function is impaired.[9] However, the previous apprehension of inducing hepatic encephalopathy with high-protein diets due to hyperammonemia from protein deamination has been put to rest. Protein restriction should not be prescribed as it increases protein catabolism and sarcopenia.[26]

Caloric intake is often reduced in cirrhosis whereas metabolic demand is high in those with advanced disease. However, in patients with cirrhosis who also have obesity, increased energy intake is not recommended; in fact, weight reduction through lifestyle interventions is recommended for those individuals due to its beneficial effect on portal hypertension. In individuals who are malnourished and have muscle depletion, current recommendations by the European Society for Clinical Nutrition and Metabolism (ESPEN) are a daily caloric intake of 30 to 35 kcal/kg of dry weight and

1.5 g of protein/kg/d. Furthermore, it is recommended that nonmalnourished patients with compensated cirrhosis consume 1.2 g of protein/kg/d. If nutritional requirements cannot be met by oral nutrition alone (**Table 11**) or in combination with oral nutrition supplements, then enteral nutrition is required. Parenteral nutrition should be used in cirrhotic patients in whom oral and enteral nutrition are ineffective or not possible.[26]

Specific Amino Acids and Hepatic Encephalopathy

The effect of specific amino acids on hepatic encephalopathy has been a topic of interest. Specifically, the branched-chain amino acids (BCAA) isoleucine, leucine, and valine, as well as the aromatic amino acids (AAA) tyrosine and phenylalanine, and their ratios have been examined. The abnormal amino acid pattern, decreased BCAA concentrations combined with elevated concentrations of AAA, has been termed the "Fischer's ratio". This ratio has been associated with the grade of hepatic encephalopathy.[27] Most interventions for patients with hepatic encephalopathy are directed at reducing blood ammonia levels, and it is believed that the beneficial effect of BCAA is associated with ammonia detoxification outside the liver, predominantly in skeletal muscles.[28] Therefore, it has been assumed that external replenishment of BCAA via the diet can have a beneficial effect on ammonia levels.[29] "Protein intolerance" is rare; however, if the cirrhosis patient develops encephalopathy when ingesting normal amounts of mixed protein, a vegetable protein diet may be beneficial since AAAs are high in meat products. BCAA-enriched formulas have been demonstrated to improve survival in severely malnourished patients with cirrhosis and improve mental state in a select group of protein intolerant encephalopathic cirrhosis patients. However, lack of reimbursement and palatability may affect patient compliance.[26]

Additional Recommendations

- Periods of starvation should be kept short by consuming 3 to 5 meals a day and a late evening snack to improve total body protein status.[26]
- Regarding sodium, balance diet palatability with the moderate advantage reducing sodium has on treating ascites due to the increased risk of lower food intake.
- Depletion of potassium, magnesium, phosphate, and other intracellular minerals frequently occurs and should be replaced.
- Deficiency in water-soluble vitamins, mainly group B vitamins, should be anticipated and treated as patients are especially at risk for developing thiamine deficiency and refeeding syndrome.
- Deficiency in fat-soluble vitamins has also been observed. If confirmed or clinically suspected, deficiencies should be treated.

FAT

Lipids can be of animal or plant origin. Their primary function is to provide cellular fuel as by weight they contain twice as much energy as protein and carbohydrate and their storage is unlimited. However, they also protect vital organs, insulate the body, produce and regulate hormones, facilitate the transport of fat-soluble vitamins, constitute vital components of cell membranes, provide essential nutrients, and contribute to satiety.[6] The three main types of dietary lipids are triglycerides, phospholipids, and sterols. Triglycerides make up more than 95% of dietary lipids, whereas phospholipids comprise approximately 2% and sterols 3%. Triglycerides and phospholipids are found in animal and plant sources whereas dietary sterols are only from animal

Table 11
Protein content of common foods

Meat, Poultry, Fish	Portion Size	Grams of Protein
Beef/turkey jerky	1 oz dried	10–15
Beef, chicken, turkey, pork, lamb	1 oz	7
Fish, tuna fish	1 oz	7
Seafood (crabmeat, shrimp, lobster)	1 oz	6
Egg	1	6
Soy and Vegetable Protein	*Portion Size*	*Grams of Protein*
Soy milk	8 oz	7
Edamame, dry roasted	1 oz	13
Tofu	1 oz	3
Legumes and Nuts	*Portion Size*	*Grams of Protein*
Lentils	½ cup	9
Lima beans	½ cup	7
Kidney, black, navy, Cannellini beans	½ cup	8
Hummus	$^1/_3$ cup	7
Chili with beans, drained	½ cup	10
Peanut butter	2 tbsp	7
Nuts	1 oz ($^1/_4$ cup)	4–6
Sunflower seeds	1 oz	5
Almond milk	8 oz	1
Milk and Dairy	*Portion Size*	*Grams of Protein*
Milk, skim, or 1%	8 oz	8
High protein ultrafiltered milk, fat-free or 1%	8 oz	13
Yogurt, fat-free, light	6 oz	5
Greek yogurt, plain, nonfat, light	5 oz	12–18
Cheese, hard (low fat)	1 oz	7
American cheese (low fat)	1 slice (0.7 oz)	5
Cottage cheese, Ricotta (part-skimmed)	½ cup	14
Grains and Cereals	*Portion Size*	*Grams of Protein*
Bread	1 oz slice	3
Cereal	½ cup hot $^3/_4$ cup cold	3
High-protein cereals	$^3/_4$-1$^1/_3$ cup	7–15
Rice, pasta	$^1/_3$ cup	3
Quinoa	$^1/_3$ cup	6
Vegetables	*Portion Size*	*Grams of Protein*
Fresh, frozen, canned	½ cup, 1 cup raw leafy greens	2
Fruit	*Portion Size*	*Grams of Protein*
Fresh or canned fruit	1 small, ½ cup	0

Johns Hopkins Medicine: https://www.hopkinsmedicine.org/bariatrics/_documents/nutrition_protein_content_common_foods.pdf.

sources.[8] The terms fats, oils, and triglycerides can be used interchangeably, and in this article, "fat" refers to triglycerides.

Triglycerides are composed of three fatty acids and a glycerol. Fatty acids can be saturated or unsaturated. The fatty acid is considered saturated if there are only single bonds between neighboring carbons in the hydrocarbon chain. The fatty acid is deemed unsaturated when the hydrocarbon chain contains a double bond. Unsaturated fats can be categorized into monounsaturated fatty acids (MUFA) and polyunsaturated fatty acids (PUFA) based on the number of double bonds. If there is a singular double bond in the molecule, it is a MUFA, and if there is more than one double bond, it is a PUFA. Most unsaturated fats are usually of plant origin, liquid at room temperature, and called oils. Fatty acids can also differ in length and be considered short chain, medium chain, or long chain based on the number of carbons. Oils are usually short chain, and animal sources are typically long chain and solid at room temperature.[6]

Many foods naturally contain fats, including dairy products, meats, poultry, seafood, and eggs, seeds, nuts, avocados, and coconuts (**Box 1**).

Box 1
Sources of dietary fat[30]

- *Saturated fats* are found in the greatest amounts in butter, beef fat, and coconut, palm, and palm kernel oils. Higher-fat meats, dairy, cakes, cookies, and some snack foods are higher in saturated fats. Dishes with many ingredients are common sources of saturated fat, including pizza, casseroles, burgers, tacos, and sandwiches.

- *Monounsaturated fats* are found in the greatest amounts in canola, olive, peanut, sunflower, and safflower oils and avocados, peanut butter, and most nuts.

- *Polyunsaturated fats* are found in the greatest amounts in sunflower, corn, soybean, and cottonseed oils and fatty fish, walnuts, and some seeds.

Clinical Relevance: Dietary Fat Composition

The American Heart Association concluded strongly that lowering the intake of saturated fat and replacing it with unsaturated fats, especially polyunsaturated fats, will reduce the incidence of cardiovascular disease. Conversely, the replacement of saturated fat with mostly refined carbohydrates and sugars does not have a beneficial effect on cardiovascular disease.[31] As a result, one of the key recommendations of the Dietary Guidelines for Americans, 2020 to 2025 is to limit saturated fat to less than 10% of calories per day starting at age 2.[2] *Trans* fats have also been implicated in coronary artery disease. To create *trans* fat, unsaturated fats (oils) are artificially hydrogenated to make them semi-solid and a desirable consistency for processed food. Doing so changes a healthy unsaturated fat to an unhealthy one.[8,32] As a result, partially hydrogenated oils, the primary source of artificial *trans* fat in the diet, are considered a health hazard and can no longer be added to foods.[2] However, since a small amount of *trans* fats can occur naturally in meat and dairy, food labels are required to display *trans* fat content.

Essential and Nonessential Fatty Acids

Fatty acids that the body can synthesize from food are known as nonessential fatty acids. However, there are some fatty acids that the body cannot synthesize, and these are considered essential fatty acids. The essential fatty acids omega-3 and omega-6 are PUFAs and must be obtained from food. Essential fatty acids are important

> **Box 2**
> **Sources of omega-3 and omega-6 fatty acids[31,33]**
>
> - *Omega 6 Sources:* safflower, sunflower, corn, sesame, soybean, and sesame oil
> - *Omega 3 Sources:* salmon, herring, sardines, lake trout, and Atlantic or Pacific mackerel, eggs (if given feed that is high in omega-3s), and ground flaxseed or flaxseed oil

structural components of cell membranes, essential for central nervous system function, play critical roles in immune and inflammatory responses, and regulate gene expression.[8] Omega-6 fatty acids, specifically linoleic acid, are more prevalent in the diet (**Box 2**). There are controversies surrounding its effects; thus, nutrition education has focused on increasing dietary intake of the omega-3 fatty acids alpha-linolenic, docosahexaenoic acid, and eicosapentaenoic acid.

The high omega-3 content of fatty fish and its benefits are underscored by the American Heart Association, concluding in a report published in 2018 that 1 to 2 seafood meals per week be included to reduce the risk of congestive heart failure, coronary heart disease, ischemic stroke, and sudden cardiac death, especially when seafood replaces the intake of less healthy foods.[33]

Clinical Relevance: Gastrointestinal Disorders Associated with Fat Metabolism

Gastroparesis

Gastroparesis is a motility disorder of the stomach that results in delayed emptying without evidence of obstruction. While idiopathic is the most common form, the majority of other causes include diabetes, medication-induced, or postsurgical.[34] The most common symptoms of gastroparesis are nausea, vomiting, early satiety, postprandial fullness, abdominal pain, and bloating.[35] These associated symptoms can negatively affect a patient's quality of life; therefore, various treatments have been developed that include dietary, medical, endoscopic, and surgical.[36] While diet is the first line treatment for gastroparesis, advice has previously been based on common sense. However, recent studies have focused on meal composition and specific trigger foods enabling practitioners to provide more evidence-based advice. Additionally, many patients with gastroparesis consume diets deficient in calories, carbohydrates, protein, vitamins, and minerals, underscoring the need for nutrition counseling.[37]

Foods that are fatty, acidic, spicy, and roughage-based have been found to increase overall symptoms in individuals with gastroparesis.[38,39] Furthermore, provoking foods were found to contain, on average, 6.5 g of fat per 100 g serving.[38] Fat slows gastric emptying, and insoluble fiber requires adequate interdigestive antral motility that is frequently absent in patients who have significantly delayed gastric emptying.

> **Box 3**
> **Patient education to reduce fat intake**
>
> - Choose low-fat or fat-free dairy products
> - Choose lean meats and trim the skin and excess fat
> - Bake, broil, and grill rather than fry
> - Limit processed foods
> - Include plenty of fruits and vegetables
> - Read all food labels

Therefore, patients should be instructed to consume a low-fat diet that is also low in insoluble fiber (**Box 3**). Patients should also be instructed to consume four to five small meals a day rather than less frequent larger meals.[34] It should be noted that liquids empty more readily than solids; however, patients should be instructed to avoid carbonated beverages since they increase gastric distention.[34,39]

SUMMARY

Following a healthy dietary pattern throughout the lifespan is vital to achieving and maintaining good health and reducing the risk of chronic disease. Nutrition is the first line of treatment and prevention of commonly encountered medical conditions and patients often seek nutrition advice from their medical providers, which underscores the need for knowledge in this area. To provide effective nutrition counseling, a clinician must have a solid foundation in knowledge of the nutrients. This article introduces the macronutrients: carbohydrate, protein, and fat and their association with commonly encountered gastrointestinal disorders. However, it should be noted that there are numerous other gastrointestinal disorders where diet and lifestyle are vital components of a patient's care plan but were beyond the scope of this article. Additionally, there is an important difference between advising patients on the basics and the in-depth counseling provided by an RDN who has the knowledge and skills to help individuals initiate and sustain a healthy dietary practice. Nutrition counseling is within a physician's and advanced practice provider's scope of practice and should be incorporated into their day-to-day patient care, but for patients with more complex issues it is essential that RDNs be included on the healthcare team.

CLINICS CARE POINTS

- Due to its health benefits, adults should consume 25 to 35 g of fiber a day or 14 g/1000 calories as per the Dietary Guidelines for Americans.
- People with celiac disease can safely consume oats uncontaminated by wheat, barley, and rye; doing so will add diversity and offer many nutritional benefits to the gluten-free diet.
- FODMAPs are fermentable short-chain carbohydrates found in everyday foods. A low FODMAP diet is implemented in three phases. The third is a maintenance phase where the patient adheres to a long-term personalized modified diet with as few restrictions as possible.
- The requirement for dietary protein correlates with growth rate and is highest in infancy and lowest in adults, 0.8 g/kg/d. However, in individuals with cirrhosis, protein recommendations range from 1.2 to 1.5 g of protein/kg/d.
- Foods that are fatty, acidic, spicy, and roughage-based have been found to increase overall symptoms in individuals with gastroparesis. Specifically, provoking foods were found to contain, on average, 6.5 g of fat per 100 g serving. Therefore, patients should be instructed to consume a low-fat diet that is also low in insoluble fiber.

DISCLOSURE

The authors have nothing to disclose.

REFERENCES

1. Centers for Disease Control and Prevention. Poor Nutrition. Available at: https://www.cdc.gov/chronicdisease/pdf/factsheets/poor-nutrition-H.pdf. Accessed November 21, 2021.

2. U.S. Department of Agriculture and U.S. Department of Health and Human Services. Dietary Guidelines for Americans, 2020-2025. 9th Edition. Available at:DietaryGuidelines.gov. Accessed November 21, 2021.

3. Green S, Shallal K. Nutrition essentials. Tempe, Arizona: Maricopa Community Colleges; 2020.

4. Merk Manuals Professional Edition. Overview of Nutrition - Nutritional Disorders. Available at: https://www.merckmanuals.com/professional/nutritional-disorders/nutrition-general-considerations/overview-of-nutrition?query=Carbohydrates,%20Proteins,%20and%20Fats. Accessed November 21, 2021.

5. Panel on Macronutrients, Panel on the Definition of Dietary Fiber, Subcommittee on Upper Reference Levels of Nutrients, et al. Dietary reference intakes for energy, carbohydrate, fiber, fat, fatty acids, cholesterol, protein, and amino acids. National Academies Press; 2005. p. 10490. https://doi.org/10.17226/10490.

6. Wakim S, Mandeep G. Human biology. Butte College; 2022. Available at: https://bio.libretexts.org/@go/page/16710.4.2. Accessed April 4, 2022.

7. Drewnowski A. Defining Nutrient Density: Development and Validation of the Nutrient Rich Foods Index. J Am Coll Nutr 2009;28(4):421S–6S. https://doi.org/10.1080/07315724.2009.10718106.

8. Calabrese A, Gibby C, Meinke B, et al. Human nutrition. University of Hawaii at Manoa; 2018. Available at: https://open.umn.edu/opentextbooks/textbooks/622. Accessed November 21, 2021.

9. Katz DL, Friedman RSC, Lucan SC. Nutrition in clinical practice: a comprehensive, evidence-based manual for the practitioner. 3rd edition. Philadelphia, Pennsylvania: Wolters Kluwer; 2015.

10. Mudgil D, Barak S. Composition, properties and health benefits of indigestible carbohydrate polymers as dietary fiber: a review. Int J Biol Macromol 2013; 61:1–6.

11. Ludvigsson JF, Leffler DA, Bai JC, et al. The Oslo definitions for coeliac disease and related terms. Gut 2013;62(1):43–52.

12. Kupper C. Dietary guidelines and implementation for celiac disease. Gastroenterology 2005;128(4):S121–7.

13. North American Society for the Study of Celiac Disease. NASSCD Releases Summary Statement on Oats. 2016. Available at: https://celiac.org/about-the-foundation/featured-news/2016/04/nasscd-releases-summary-statement-on-oats/. Accessed November 24, 2021.

14. Food and Drug Administration. Gluten-Free Labeling of Foods. 2020. https://www.fda.gov/food/food-labeling-nutrition/gluten-free-labeling-foods. [Accessed 24 November 2021]. Accessed.

15. Lovell RM, Ford AC. Global prevalence of and risk factors for irritable bowel syndrome: a meta-analysis. Clin Gastroenterol Hepatol 2012;10:712–21.

16. Ford AC, Moayyedi P, Chey WD, et al. American college of gastroenterology monograph on management of irritable bowel syndrome. Am J Gastroenterol 2018;113(Suppl 2):1–18.

17. Motl A, Vakil N. FODMAPS Everywhere and not a Thing to Eat. Pract Gastroenterol 2019;118:33–41.

18. Riby JE, Fujisawa T, Kretchmer N. Fructose absorption. Am J Clin Nutr 1993;58(5 Suppl):748S–53S.

19. Rao SSC, Attaluri A, Anderson L, et al. Ability of the normal human small intestine to absorb fructose: evaluation by breath testing. Clin Gastroenterol Hepatol 2007; 5(8):959–63.

20. Truswell AS, Seach JM, Thorburn AW. Incomplete absorption of pure fructose in healthy subjects and the facilitating effect of glucose. Am J Clin Nutr 1988;48(6): 1424–30.
21. Deng Y, Misselwitz B, Dai N, et al. Lactose intolerance in adults: biological mechanism and dietary management. Nutrients 2015;7(9):8020–35.
22. Itan Y, Jones BL, Ingram CJE, et al. A worldwide correlation of lactase persistence phenotype and genotypes. BMC Evol Biol 2010;10:36.
23. Shaukat A, Levitt MD, Taylor BC, et al. Systematic review: effective management strategies for lactose intolerance. Ann Intern Med 2010;152(12):797–803.
24. Varney J, Barrett J, Scarlata K, et al. FODMAPs: food composition, defining cutoff values and international application: Defining and adapting the low-FODMAP diet. J Gastroenterol Hepatol 2017;32:53–61.
25. Staudacher HM, Rossi M, Kaminski T, et al. Long-term personalized low FODMAP diet improves symptoms and maintains luminal Bifidobacteria abundance in irritable bowel syndrome. Neurogastroenterol Motil 2021. https://doi.org/10.1111/nmo.14241.
26. Bischoff SC, Bernal W, Dasarathy S, et al. Espen practical guideline: clinical nutrition in liver disease. Clin Nutr 2020;39(12):3533–62.
27. Fischer JE, Rosen HM, Ebeid AM, et al. The effect of normalization of plasma amino acids on hepatic encephalopathy in man. Surgery 1976;80(1):77–91.
28. Tajiri K. Branched-chain amino acids in liver diseases. World J Gastroenterol 2013;19(43):7620.
29. Dam G, Aamann L, Vistrup H, et al. The role of Branched Chain Amino Acids in the treatment of hepatic Encephalopathy. J Clin Exp Hepatol 2018;8(4):448–51.
30. National Institute on Aging. Important Nutrients to Know: Proteins, Carbohydrates, and Fats. Available at: http://www.nia.nih.gov/health/important-nutrients-know-proteins-carbohydrates-and-fats. Accessed January 1, 2022.
31. Sacks FM, Lichtenstein AH, Wu JHY, et al. Dietary fats and cardiovascular disease: a presidential advisory from the american heart association. Circulation 2017;136(3). https://doi.org/10.1161/CIR.0000000000000510.
32. Marchand V. Trans fats: What physicians should know. Paediatr Child Health 2010;15(6):373–8.
33. Rimm EB, Appel LJ, Chiuve SE, et al. Seafood long-chain n-3 polyunsaturated fatty acids and cardiovascular disease: a science advisory from the american heart association. Circulation 2018;138(1). https://doi.org/10.1161/CIR.0000000000000574.
34. Camilleri M, Parkman HP, Shafi MA, et al. Clinical guideline: management of gastroparesis. Am J Gastroenterol 2013;108(1):18–37 [quiz: 38].
35. Revicki DA, Camilleri M, Kuo B, et al. Development and content validity of a gastroparesis cardinal symptom index daily diary. Aliment Pharmacol Ther 2009; 30(6):670–80.
36. Camilleri M. Novel Diet, Drugs, and Gastric Interventions for Gastroparesis. Clin Gastroenterol Hepatol 2016;14(8):1072–80.
37. Parkman HP, Yates KP, Hasler WL, et al. Dietary intake and nutritional deficiencies in patients with diabetic or idiopathic gastroparesis. Gastroenterology 2011; 141(2):486–98, 498.e1-7.
38. Wytiaz V, Homko C, Duffy F, et al. Foods provoking and alleviating symptoms in gastroparesis: patient experiences. Dig Dis Sci 2015;60(4):1052–8.
39. Homko CJ, Duffy F, Friedenberg FK, et al. Effect of dietary fat and food consistency on gastroparesis symptoms in patients with gastroparesis. Neurogastroenterol Motil 2015;27(4):501–8.

Decoding Plant-Based and Other Popular Diets
Ensuring Patients Are Meeting Their Nutrient Needs

Christine Werner, PhD, PA-C, RDN[a],*, Elaina Osterbur, PhD[b]

KEYWORDS

- Plant-based diets • Lacto-ovo-vegetarian • Lacto-vegetarian • Pescatarian • Vegan
- Mediterranean • Paleo • Intermittent fasting

KEY POINTS

- Vegetarianism and varying patterns of vegetarian diets are considered safe and nutritious with appropriate meal planning.
- Attention to vegetarian food sources for specific nutrients such as calcium, iron, Vitamin B12 and Vitamin D needs to be prioritized to prevent risk of select nutrient deficiencies.
- The Mediterranean diet is the easiest diet to follow with careful portion-controlled meal planning to prevent excess caloric intake.
- The Paleo diet may promote the overconsumption of meat and over time lack dietary calcium and Vitamin D that would need to be addressed to prevent nutrient deficiencies.
- Intermittent fasting can be a safe and effective diet but is not recommended for some at-risk groups that include children and teens under the age of 18, women who are pregnant or breastfeeding, individuals with kidney stones, gastroesophageal reflux, and diabetes.

BACKGROUND

The majority (72%) of Americans agree that a healthy diet is important to their overall long-term well-being.[1] A healthy diet aids in growth and longer life, and lowers the risks of certain cancers, obesity, type 2 diabetes, heart disease, and stroke.[2] Further research suggests that diets lower in animal foods and higher in plant foods are among the healthiest.[3] These diets include vegan, vegetarian, and Mediterranean.[3] Approximately 3.3% of American adults identify as vegan or vegetarian.[4] Approximately 3% of

The authors have nothing to disclose.
[a] Physician Assistant Program, Department of Clinical Health Sciences, Saint Louis University, DCHS, Suite 3082, 3437 Caroline Street, St Louis, MO 63104, USA; [b] Program in Health Sciences, Department of Clinical Health Sciences, Saint Louis University, DCHS, Suite 3025, 3437 Caroline Street, St Louis, MO 63104, USA
* Corresponding author.
E-mail address: christine.werner@health.slu.edu

Physician Assist Clin 7 (2022) 615–628
https://doi.org/10.1016/j.cpha.2022.05.002
2405-7991/22/© 2022 Elsevier Inc. All rights reserved.

Americans follow a Paleo diet whereas 5% and 9% follow the Mediterranean and intermittent fasting diets, respectively.[4,5]

VEGETARIAN DIETS

A vegetarian may be defined as lacto-ovo-vegetarian, lacto-vegetarian, semivegetarian, pescatarian, or vegan.[5,6] A lacto-vegetarian dietary pattern includes dairy (products containing milk or made from milk) products as well as plant-based foods. A lacto-ovo-vegetarian diet includes eggs and dairy with a plant-based diet. A semivegetarian diet includes plant-based foods and small amounts of animal protein (dairy, poultry, fish), excluding red meat. A pescatarian diet adds fish to a plant-based diet and a vegan is restricted to plant-based sources alone excluding all animal proteins and animal by-products (dairy, eggs, honey, gelatin, etc.). Regardless of vegetarian diet preference, it is universally recommended that individuals choose a variety of food categories or groups to ensure adequate nutrient needs are met over time.[4]

Benefits

Vegetarianism is a socially accepted diet and is supported by the American Institute for Cancer Research, The National School Lunch Program, and the US Department of Agriculture. The Academy of Nutrition and Dietetics supports a vegetarian diet pattern, including vegan diets that are appropriately planned. The Academy of Nutrition and Dietetics suggests that vegetarian diets are appropriate for all stages of life, including pregnancy, lactation, infancy, childhood, adolescence, older adulthood, and for athletes, yet stresses the importance of a carefully planned diet.[5] Research suggests that when a vegetarian diet is consistently followed it can prevent and treat certain diseases.[4] Vegetarians and vegans are at a reduced risk of type 2 diabetes, hypertension, heart disease, obesity, and some cancers.[4] Vegetarian and vegan diets are lower in saturated fats as well as rich in fiber that can lower cholesterol and serum glucose levels.[4]

Risks

The Academy of Nutrition and Dietetics agrees there are specific dietary nutrients a strict plant-based diet (vegan) lacks such as protein, calcium, iron, Vitamin B12, and Vitamin D, and extra care should be taken to ensure they are incorporated in meal planning schemes.[4]

Protein

Dietary protein is made up of different amino acids that play a role in the growth and maintenance of all body cells and tissues, along with enzyme, antibody, and hormone production. There are 20 different amino acids bonded together to form a protein. Out of these 20, 11 amino acids are synthesized within the human body (nonessential) whereas the remaining 9 amino acids require dietary consumption (essential), to obtain adequate protein intake.[7] A protein source is considered "complete" when it contains all 9 essential amino acids whereas "incomplete" protein foods contain some, but not all the essential amino acids.[7]

Examples of "complete" proteins include fish, poultry, eggs, beef, pork, dairy products, soy products (ie, soy milk, tofu, edamame, tempeh, miso), and hemp milk. "Incomplete" proteins include beans, peas, lentils, nuts, seeds, whole grains, and vegetables (**Table 1**).

Historically, adequate protein intake in a vegetarian diet with no animal products has been a concern. However, evidence over the years suggests that the consistent daily consumption of plant-based foods and in variety can achieve or exceed the

Table 1
Semivegetarian options for protein sources

Complete Proteins	Incomplete Proteins
Fish	Beans
Poultry	Peas
Eggs	Lentils
Beef	Nuts
Pork	Seeds
Dairy products	Whole grains
Soy products (soy milk, tofu, edamame, tempeh, miso) and hemp milk	Vegetables

recommended protein intake in strict vegetarians or vegans when caloric intake is sufficient to meet energy needs.[6,8]

The daily consumption of plant-based foods such as soy, certain plant-based milks, meat substitutes, legumes (peas, beans, and lentils), nuts, nut butter and whole grains can assure sufficient total protein needs, without the need to combine specific foods together, at a given meal.[6,8]

Calcium
Adequate calcium intake is essential for bone health, neuromuscular functioning, and blood coagulation, among other physiologic roles in the human body.[6] The recommended dietary allowance (RDA) for calcium, for most adults, is between 1000 to 1200 mg/d[6] Milk and dairy products contain the highest concentration of calcium in each food serving.[9] Vegetarians and vegans who depend on plant-based foods are at risk of calcium deficiency. Individuals on plant-based diets can explore a variety of nondairy fortified commercial food products such as various kinds of milk (almond, oat, soy), tofu, or ready-to-eat cereals. In addition, nuts, beans, legumes, and specific leafy green vegetables are good plant-based calcium sources (**Table 2**). Due to the variety of plant-based commercial food products on the market, it is advised to review the specific food labels for nutrient content per serving.[9]

Table 2
Vegetarian options for calcium sources

Fortified options for commercial plant-based foods	Milks—almond, oats, soy Tofu Juices Ready-to-eat cereals Butters—almond, tahini
Green vegetables	Collard greens Kale Bok choy Broccoli
Beans, nuts	Soybeans Chickpeas Black beans Chili beans Almonds

Calcium absorption from plant foods varies due to the concentration of phytic acid, highest in grains and legumes, consumed during the same meal. Oxalic acids, which are particularly high in plant foods such as beets, spinach, and Swiss chard can also impede calcium absorption.[4] Boiling may reduce the amount of oxalic acid in various leafy green vegetables and soaking grains overnight may reduce their phytic acid although it is unclear if the degree of calcium absorption significantly changes.[8]

Iron

Iron is considered an essential mineral responsible for the production of oxygen transport proteins such as hemoglobin and myoglobin, DNA synthesis, and electron transport.[10] Heme iron (animal source) is reported to have higher absorption rates (15%–30%) than nonheme (plant-based) iron (5%–10%) sources.[8] Vegetarian diets that incorporate a variety of different plant-based iron sources can reduce the risk of iron deficiency anemia.[8] The recommended dietary allowance (RDA) for iron, for most adults, is 8 mg/day[10] (**Table 3**).

The absorption of iron (nonheme) from plants and plant-based foods is reported to vary based on the presence of multiple dietary components including the presence of Vitamin C, other organic acids, and inhibitors like phytates.[8] Additionally, the absorption of nonheme iron is demonstrated to be inversely related to the iron status of the individual.[4] Humans with low iron stores absorb greater degrees of iron whereas those with adequate iron stores absorb less iron to avoid iron overload.[4]

Vitamin B12

Vitamin B12 (cobalamin) is a water-soluble vitamin required for proper red blood cell formation, nerve development and function, and DNA synthesis.[11] Vitamin B12

Table 3 Plant-based options for iron	
Fortified Options	**Plant Milks (Check Label)**
Green vegetables	Collard greens Kale Spinach Broccoli
Dried fruits	Prunes Raisins Apricots
Beans and legumes	White, lima, navy beans White/red kidney beans Black-eyed peas Lentils Chickpeas Soybeans Tofu Tempeh Natto
Nuts, seeds	Sesame Pumpkin Flaxseeds Hemp seeds
Other sources	Black-strap molasses

deficiency can develop through dietary deficiency, lack of intrinsic factor, history of gastric or ileal resection, ileitis, and certain congenital conditions.[11] Vitamin B12 deficiency can cause megaloblastic anemia along with physical and neurologic signs and symptoms that may become irreversible.[11] Vitamin B12 absorption requires a glycoprotein, called the "intrinsic factor", produced by the parietal cells in the lining of the stomach. It attaches to B12, and then the B12 is transported to the terminal ileum of the small intestine where it is absorbed.[11]

The RDA for Vitamin B12, for most adults, is 2.4 mcg/day.[11] Because the intrinsic factor protein becomes saturated at about half the RDA, B12 absorption requires 4 to 6 hours.[4] Because of this phenomenon, it has been recommended to consume Vitamin B12 rich foods at least twice a day, to optimize absorption.[4] When ingesting large supplemental doses of Vitamin B12 approximately 1% of the dose is absorbed by passive diffusion.[8]

Vitamin B12 is naturally present in animal foods including beef, poultry, eggs, fish, and dairy products. Plants and plant-based foods do not contain Vitamin B12 unless the product is fortified with Vitamin B12.[11] Unlike other water-soluble vitamins, Vitamin B12 is stored in the liver and a deficiency may take years to develop as a result of prolonged inadequate consumption. Individuals adhering to strict vegan practices (no animal, eggs, or dairy products), should consume at least two vitamin-fortified foods like plant-based milks, cereals and/or soy products[4] (**Table 4**). Individuals who lack intrinsic factor, have had a gastric or ileal resection, or have ileitis should supplement B12 sublingually, bypassing the GI tract.

Vitamin D

Vitamin D, a fat-soluble vitamin, promotes calcium absorption from the gut and maintains adequate serum calcium and phosphate concentrations to regulate bone mineralization.[12] Vitamin D also plays a role in the reduction of inflammation, modulation of cell growth, and neuromuscular and immune function.[12] In addition to dietary sources, it is also produced endogenously via direct skin sunlight exposure. Obtaining adequate cutaneous Vitamin D is dependent on several factors including skin pigmentation, sunscreen use, time of day, latitude, altitude, air pollution, clothing over the skin, and aging.[4,12]

The recommended dietary allowance (RDA) for Vitamin D, for most adults, is 600 IU/day[13] (**Table 5**). Over age 70, the RDA is 700 IU/day. Vitamin D is naturally present in animal-based foods, and in a few plant-based foods in lower concentrations, if not fortified. Individuals adhering to a strict vegan food pattern (no animal-based foods) should consume at least two Vitamin D fortified plant-based foods; if not include a daily supplement meeting the RDA[4,14]

Table 4 Vitamin B12 options for Lacto-ovo-vegetarians	
Source	mcg Per Serving
Egg, whole, cooked, 1 large	0.5
Milk, 2%, 1 cup	1.3
Fortified breakfast cereals (check label)	0.6
Nutritional yeast, fortified (check label), ¼ cup	8.3–2.4
Fortified plant-based milk (check label)	
Tempeh, ½ cup	0.1

Table 5
Vitamin D options for Lacto-ovo-vegetarians and pescatarians

Source	IU Per Serving
Egg, whole, cooked, 1 large	44
Milk, 2%, Vitamin D fortified 1 cup	120
Fortified breakfast cereals (check label)	80
Fortified Vitamin D orange juice (check label)	~100
Fortified plant-based milk (check label), 1 cup	100–144
Mushrooms, white, raw, exposed to UV light, ½ Cup	0.1
Trout, rainbow (farmed, 3 oz. cooked)	645
Salmon (farmed)	240
Salmon (wild)	988
Canned tuna, mackerel, and sardines (packed in water)	240

Recommendations

Vegetarian diets that exclude dairy products and animal proteins may lack dietary nutrients such as calcium, iron, Vitamin B12, and Vitamin D. Careful meal planning that includes nondairy calcium sources, and Vitamin B12- and Vitamin D-fortified commercial products such as plant-based milks (almond, oats, soy), tofu, and cereals or supplements can aid in meeting the RDA of these vital nutrients. Iron from plant-based sources alone may not meet an individual's RDA requirements and an iron supplement may be warranted. Clinicians should educate their patients on the importance of these nutrients to their health. Furthermore, they should refer their vegan patients to a registered dietitian (RD) for individualized education to ensure they are meeting their nutrient needs.

MEDITERRANEAN DIET
Background

The Mediterranean diet is one of the most researched diets in the world.[15] It was first discovered among cultures in geographic areas of olive cultivation along the Mediterranean coast.[15,16] It is focused on the high intake of fruits, vegetables, nuts, grains, olive oil, moderate intake of dairy products, low-to-moderate intake of fish, and low intake of red meat and wine (**Fig. 1**).[15–17] The diet has been associated with longer life expectancy and lower rates of chronic disease.[15,18,19] It is also recommended by the American Heart Association (AHA) because it achieves the AHA's recommendations for a healthy dietary pattern.[20]

Benefits

The Mediterranean diet can prevent heart disease and stroke by reducing risk factors such as obesity, diabetes, high cholesterol, and high blood pressure. Furthermore, some studies suggest that diets rich in virgin olive oil may help the body remove excess cholesterol from arteries.[20] Studies suggest that adherence to a Mediterranean diet leads to the prevention of chronic diseases including diabetes, cardiovascular disease, some cancers, and mental health conditions[18] (**Table 6**). Furthermore, studies suggest that the Mediterranean diet can increase life expectancy.[15,18,19] The Nurses' Health study suggests that women ages 57 to 61 who followed a Mediterranean-type diet were 46% more likely to experience healthy aging. Healthy aging as defined is living to 70 years or more, having no chronic disease or

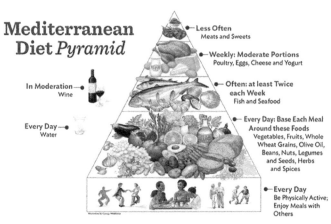

Fig. 1. Mediterranean diet pyramid. (From: Oldways Preservation and Exchange Trust. Available at Mediterranean Diet | Oldways (oldwayspt.org) Accessed February 2022.)

major declines in mental health, cognition, and physical function. The increased intake of plant foods, whole grains, and fish; moderate alcohol consumption; and low intake of red and processed meats were believed to contribute to this finding.[28] Another important benefit is that the Mediterranean diet is the easiest diet to follow.[29]

Risks

There is the potential risk of excess calorie intake because the diet does not specify portions and includes fats from olive oil and nuts.[20] The Mediterranean diet is lower in consumption of meats and carbohydrates than a traditional American diet.[30,31] Therefore, the risk of lower iron consumption exists so diets should include foods rich in iron and Vitamin C which aids in iron absorption.[32] Fewer dairy products are consumed in the Mediterranean diet; therefore, calcium loss could occur. Clinicians should be cognizant of their patient's need for calcium supplementation.[32] The Mediterranean diet also recommends the consumption of wine. However, wine should not be consumed by individuals who are pregnant, prone to alcohol abuse, or at risk of

Table 6
Mediterranean diet prescription for prevention

Condition	Current Population Morbidity Rates
Cancer	9.5%[21]
High cholesterol	20.1%[22]
Hypertension	27.0%[23]
Heart attack/myocardial infarction	3.1%[24]
Chronic obstructive pulmonary disease (COPD)/emphysema chronic bronchitis	4.6%[25]
Arthritis	21.4%[26]
Regularly had feelings of worry, nervousness, or anxiety	11.1%[27]

Conditions that the Mediterranean diet may prevent or decrease the risk.

breast cancer.[32] Furthermore, wine consumption should not exceed the Dietary Guidelines for Americans.

Recommendations

The Mediterranean diet is the easiest diet to follow. However. because the diet does not specify portions careful meal planning is important to maintain a healthy weight. The diet should include foods rich in iron, Vitamin C, and calcium. If the RDA requirements cannot be met through careful meal planning, then nutrient supplementation should be considered.

PALEO DIET
Background

The Paleo diet is a food pattern based on the Paleolithic era, dating from approximately 2.5 million to 10,000 years ago.[33] The Paleo diet may often be referred to as the caveman diet, the Stone Age diet, Paleolithic diet, or the hunter-gatherer diet. The purpose of the Paleo diet is to eat as humans did during the Paleolithic era (**Table 7**). According to the discordance hypothesis, the human body is genetically incompatible with diets that resulted from farming practices that emerged approximately 10,000 years ago. Farming introduced dairy, grains, and legumes. The hypothesis suggests that the rapid change in diet inhibited the body's ability to adapt and this incompatibility has resulted in the prevalence of obesity, diabetes, and heart disease today.[33] Opponents of the discordance hypothesis suggest there are variations in nutritional needs based on geography, climate, and food availability and that the transition to farming has played a role in the evolution of these nutritional needs. However, studies also suggest that early human diets included grains before the introduction of farming. Furthermore, genetic research suggests that evolutionary changes continued after the Paleolithic era including the ability to digest and absorb dietary starches.[33]

The Paleo diet promotes the consumption of fruits, vegetables, and nuts, which are nutrient-dense foods, in line with the current Dietary Guidelines for Americans.[34,35] The exclusion of processed foods, refined sugar, cereals, and grains reduce caloric consumption generating greater weight loss, if weight reduction is indicated.[36]

Benefits

Several randomized clinical trials have compared the Paleo diet to other diets, such as the Mediterranean diet. The results suggest that a Paleo diet may provide some benefits such as more weight loss, improved glucose tolerance, improved blood pressure

Table 7	
The Paleo Diet's dietary inclusions and exclusions	
Inclusions	**Exclusions**
Grass-fed, free-range, or organic animal meats and wild game	Cereal grains
Fish/seafood	Legumes including peanuts
Fresh fruits	Dairy
Fresh vegetables (excluding potatoes)	Refined sugar
Eggs	Potatoes
Nuts	Processed foods
Seeds	Overly salty foods
Oils—olive, walnut, flaxseed, macadamia, avocado, coconut	Refined vegetable oils

control, lower triglycerides, and weight management. The authors of these trials caution that longer trials with larger sample sizes randomly assigned to a variety of diets should be conducted to understand the long-term, overall health benefits and risks of a Paleo Diet.[33] The Paleo diet has been associated with weight loss and other benefits.[33,33]

Studies suggest that the Paleo diet may improve or maintain blood pressure status as well as improve or maintain lipid values.[37,38] It may improve or maintain blood glucose and insulin sensitivity for diabetes as well.[38,39] It should be noted that these results are from studies in which the research designs varied, and each had small sample sizes as well as varying durations.[35,37]

Risks

The Paleo diet may over time lack dietary calcium and Vitamin D leading to an increase in osteoporosis and fractures.[35,36] The degree of meat intake, depending on the type and amount of meats consumed, can lead to an increased risk of death, cardiovascular disease, and diabetes.[36] Whole grains and legumes are high in dietary fiber, minerals, and vitamins and have their own benefits in reducing cardiovascular disease, diabetes, diverticular disease, and constipation; their absence from the diet can increase the risk of these diseases and conditions.[34,36] Additionally, the Paleo diet recommends wild game and meats that are unprocessed, grass-fed, or free-range that are not often readily available and often unaffordable.[33,34] There is a lack of long-term clinical trials identifying the benefits and risks of a Paleo food pattern.[33]

Recommendations

Many of the food sources restricted by the Paleo diet over time could result in a lack of dietary calcium and Vitamin D consumption. Furthermore, the overconsumption of meat may put the patient at risk for cardiovascular disease and diabetes. Very careful meal planning and nutrient supplementation may be recommended to meet the RDA requirements of nutrients necessary for long-term health; therefore, clinicians should consider referring patients who choose a Paleo diet to an RD.

INTERMITTENT FASTING
Background

Intermittent fasting (IF) has been defined as maintaining regular durations of no or limited caloric intake. IF also may be referred to as alternate-day fasting, reduced meal frequency, and time-restricted feeding. The most common IF dietary strategies include a daily fast for 16 hours, a 24-h fast on alternate days, or a fast 2 days per week on nonconsecutive days.[40] Studies suggest that IF leads to altered body metabolism with long-term benefits.[41] Research also suggests that IF may be more beneficial than other diets for reducing and improving conditions associated with inflammation.[42]

Benefits

Research has demonstrated that the IF diet improves conditions associated with inflammation such as Alzheimer's disease, arthritis, asthma, multiple sclerosis, and stroke.[42] A meta-analysis of randomized controlled trials suggests statistically significant improvement of body mass index, body weight, fat mass, low-density lipoprotein cholesterol, total cholesterol, triglycerides, fasting blood glucose, fasting insulin, homeostatic model assessment of insulin resistance (HOMA-IR), and blood pressure.[41] Studies also found that modified alternate-day fasting for one to 2 months was associated with a moderate reduction in body mass index in healthy adults, and adults with overweight, obesity or nonalcoholic fatty liver disease compared with a regular diet.[41]

Table 8
Examples of food portions based on a daily caloric level of 2000

Food Group	Servings Per Day
Vegetables	2 ½ cups
Fruits	2 cups
Grains	6 ½ oz
Dairy	3 cups
Protein foods	3 ½ oz
Oils	27 g (1.8 tbsp)

Calories for healthy vegetarian and Mediterranean diets.
Adapted from U.S. Department of Agriculture and U.S. Department of Health and Human Services. Dietary Guidelines for Americans. 2020-2025. 9th Edition. December 2020.

Risks

There are side effects of IF including hunger, fatigue, insomnia, nausea, and headaches.[42] IF is not recommended for children and teens under the age of 18, women who are pregnant or breast-feeding, individuals with kidney stones, gastroesophageal reflux, diabetes, or for those with a history of eating disorders.[42–44]

Recommendations

Patient health records should be consulted to determine if an intermittent fasting regime is safe for the patient. Careful fasting schedules and meal planning should be an essential part of the plan for the patient to adhere to the IF diet.

SUMMARY

All the diets reviewed have health benefits. Vegetarian and vegan dietary patterns reduce the risk of type 2 diabetes, hypertension, heart disease, obesity, and certain cancers as well as lower cholesterol and serum glucose levels. The Mediterranean diet is associated with longer life expectancy and prevention of chronic disease and certain cancers by reducing risk factors such as obesity, diabetes, high cholesterol, and high blood pressure. The Paleo diet can increase weight loss, improve glucose tolerance, and blood pressure, and lower triglycerides. The IF diet has shown to be beneficial in reducing and improving conditions associated with inflammation such as Alzheimer's disease, arthritis, multiple sclerosis, and stroke.

These diets however are not without risk. Vegetarian and vegan diets may lack the RDA requirements of calcium, iron, Vitamin B12, and Vitamin D, which can lead to osteoporosis, fractures, anemia, and physical and neurologic conditions that may not be reversible. The Mediterranean diet can result in excess caloric intake and low iron absorption which can lead to weight gain and anemia. The Paleo diet can over time lack dietary calcium and Vitamin D, which can increase the risk of osteoporosis and fractures. In general, these diets do not specify portions and lack some necessary food sources to meet RDA nutrient requirements. Therefore, a carefully planned diet is paramount for patients to maintain a healthy weight and prevent the risk of deficiency and disease (**Table 8**). Dietary supplements, as well as referral to a D, should be considered for patients choosing these dietary patterns.

CLINICS CARE POINTS

- A healthy diet aids in growth, longer life, and lowers the risk of certain cancers, obesity, type 2 diabetes, heart disease, and stroke.
- It is universally recommended that vegetarians choose a variety of food categories or groups to ensure adequate nutrient needs are met over time.
- The Mediterranean diet is recommended by the American Heart Association because it achieves its recommendation for a healthy dietary pattern.
- The Paleo diet promotes the consumption of fruits, vegetables, and nuts which are nutrient-dense foods.
- Intermittent fasting may be more beneficial than other diets for reducing and improving conditions associated with inflammation.
- A carefully planned diet is paramount for patients to maintain a healthy weight and prevent the risk of deficiency and disease. Referral to a RD may be necessary to ensure patients are meeting their nutrient needs.

REFERENCES

1. Funk C, Kennedy B. The new food fights: US public divides over food science. Washington, DC: Pew Research Center; 2016.
2. Centers for Disease Control and Prevention [CDC]. Poor Nutrition. 2020. Available at: https://www.cdc.gov/chronicdisease/resources/publications/factsheets/nutrition.htm. Accessed December 2, 2021.
3. Gan KH, Cheong HC, Tu Y, et al. Association Between Plant-Based Dietary Patterns And Risk Of Cardiovascular Disease: A Systematic Review And Meta-Analysis Of Prospective Cohort Studies. Nutrients 2021;13:3952.
4. Melina V, Craig W, Levin S. Positions of the Academy of Nutrition and Dietetics: Vegetarian Diets. J Acad Nutr Diet 2016;116(12):1970–80.
5. Vegetarian diet: how to get the best nutrition. Healthy lifestyle, nutrition and healthy eating. Rochester, MN: Mayo Clinic; 2020.
6. National Institutes of Health. Office of Dietary Supplements. Calcium. 2021. Calcium - health professional fact sheet (nih.gov). Available at: https://ods.od.nih.gov/factsheets/Calcium-HealthProfessional/. Accessed January 2022.
7. Do You Need to Worry About Eating 'Complete' Proteins. Health Essentials, Nutrition. Cleveland Clinic; 2019. Available at: from https://health.clevelandclinic.org/do-i-need-to-worry-about-eating-complete-proteins/#:~:text=Do%20you%20really%20need%20to,and%20build%20and%20repair%20tissue. Accessed Jun 20, 2022.
8. Craig WJ, Mangels AR, Fresa'n U, et al. The Safe and Effective Use of Plant-Based Diets with Guidelines for Health Professionals. Nutrients 2021;13:4144.
9. Mediterranean diet for heart health. Healthy lifestyle, nutrition and healthy eating. Rochester, MN: Mayo Clinic; 2021.
10. National Institutes of Health, Office of Dietary Supplements. Iron. 2021. Iron - Health Professional Fact Sheet (nih.gov). Available at: https://ods.od.nih.gov/factsheets/Iron-HealthProfessional/. Accessed January 2022.
11. National Institutes of Health, Office of Dietary Supplements. Vitamin B-12. 2021. Vitamin B12 - Health Professional Fact Sheet (nih.gov). Available at: https://ods.od.nih.gov/factsheets/VitaminB12-HealthProfessional/. Accessed January 2022.

12. National Institutes of Health, Office of Dietary Supplements. Vitamin D. 2021. Vitamin D - Health Professional Fact Sheet (nih.gov). Available at: https://ods.od.nih.gov/factsheets/VitaminD-HealthProfessional/. Accessed January 2022.

13. National Institutes of Health, Office of Dietary Supplements. Nutrient Recommendations: Dietary Reference Intakes. 2021. Nutrient Recommendations : Dietary Reference Intakes (DRI) (nih.gov). Available at: https://ods.od.nih.gov/HealthInformation/Dietary_Reference_Intakes.aspx. Accessed January 2022.

14. Al-Ma'aitah A, Tayyem RF. Review article vegetarian diet: health implications and nutrients' adequacy. Pakistan: Pak. J. Nutr; 2020.

15. Guasch-Ferre M, Willett WC. The mediterranean diet and health: a comprehensive overview. J Intern Med 2021;290:549–66.

16. Lăcătusu CM, Grigorescu ED, Floria M, et al. The mediterranean diet: from an environment-driven food culture to an emerging medical prescription. Int J Environ Res PU 2019;16:942.

17. Papadaki A, Nolen-Doerr E, Mantzoros CS. the effect of the mediterranean diet on metabolic health: a systematic review and meta-analysis of controlled trials in adults. Nutrients 2020;12:3342.

18. Santella ME, Hagedorn RL, Wattick RA, et al. Learn first, practice second approach to increase health professionals' nutrition-related knowledge. Attitudes and Self-Efficacy 2020;71(3):370–7.

19. Fernández AI, Bermejo J, Yotti R, et al. The impact of mediterranean diet on coronary plaque vulnerability, microvascular function, inflammation and microbiome after an acute coronary syndrome: study protocol for the MEDIMACS randomized, controlled. Mechanistic Clin Trial 2021;22:795.

20. American Heart Association. What is the Mediterranean Diet? 2020. Available at: https://www.heart.org/en/healthy-living/healthy-eating/eat-smart/nutrition-basics/mediterranean-diet. Accessed Jun 20, 2022.

21. National Center for Health Statistics. Percentage of Any Type of Cancer for Adults Aged 18 and Over, United States, 2019. National Health Interview Survey. Generated interactively. Available at: https://wwwn.cdc.gov/NHISDataQueryTool/SHS_2019_ADULT3/index.html. Accessed Jan 19, 2022.

22. National Center for Health Statistics. Percentage of High Cholesterol for Adults Aged 18 and Over, United States, 2019. National Health Interview Survey. Generated interactively. Available at: https://wwwn.cdc.gov/NHISDataQueryTool/SHS_2019_ADULT3/index.html. Accessed Jan 19, 2022.

23. National Center for Health Statistics. Diagnosed Hypertension for Adults Aged 18 and Over, United States, 2019. National Health Interview Survey. Generated interactively. Available at: https://wwwn.cdc.gov/NHISDataQueryTool/SHS_2019_ADULT3/index.html. Accessed Jan 19, 2022.

24. National Center for Health Statistics. Percentage of Heart Attack for Adults Aged 18 and Over, United States, 2019. National Health Interview Survey. Generated interactively. Available at: https://wwwn.cdc.gov/NHISDataQueryTool/SHS_2019_ADULT3/index.html. Accessed Jan 19, 2022.

25. National Center for Health Statistics. Percentage of COPD, Emphysema, or Chronic Bronchitis for Adults Aged 18 and Over, United States, 2019. National Health Interview Survey. Generated interactively. Available at: https://wwwn.cdc.gov/NHISDataQueryTool/SHS_2019_ADULT3/index.html. Accessed Jan 19, 2022.

26. National Center for Health Statistics. Percentage Of Arthritis Diagnosis for Adults Aged 18 and Over, United States, 2019. National Health Interview Survey.

Generated interactively. Available at: https://wwwn.cdc.gov/NHISDataQueryTool/SHS_2019_ADULT3/index.html. Accessed Jan 19, 2022.

27. National Center for Health Statistics. Percentage of Regularly Having Feelings of Worry, Nervousness, or Anxiety For Adults Aged 18 and Over, United States, 2019. National Health Interview Survey. Generated interactively. Available at: https://wwwn.cdc.gov/NHISDataQueryTool/SHS_2019_ADULT3/index.html. Accessed Jan 19, 2022.

28. Harvard T. H. Chan School of Public Health. The Nutrition Source. Diet Review: Mediterranean Diet. 2018. Available at: https://www.hsph.harvard.edu/nutritionsource/healthy-weight/diet-reviews/mediterranean-diet/. Accessed Jun 20, 2022.

29. Doheny K. Mediterranean Diet Repeats as Best Overall of 2020. 2020 Nourish by WebMD. Available at: https://www.webmd.com/diet/news/20200102/mediterranean-diet-repeats-as-best-overall-of-2020#:~:text=Jan.,Approaches%20to%20Stop%20Hypertension)%20diet. Accessed Jun 20, 2022.

30. National Institutes of Health. National Library of Medicine. Mediterranean Diet. 2020. Available at: https://medlineplus.gov/ency/patientinstructions/000110.htm. Accessed Jun 20, 2022.

31. Mauriello LM, Artz K. Culinary medicine: bringing healthcare into the kitchen. Am J Health Promot 2020;33(5):825–9.

32. National Institutes of Health. Mediterranean diet. Washington, DC: Medline Plus. Encyclopedia; 2020.

33. Paleo diet: what is it and why is it so popular? mayo clinic. paleo diet: what is it and why is it so popular? - mayo clinic. Available at: https://www.mayoclinic.org/healthy-lifestyle/nutrition-and-healthy-eating/in-depth/paleo-diet/art-20111182. Accessed February 2022.

34. Klemm S. Should We Eat Like Our Caveman Ancestors? Eatright.org. Academy of Nutrition and Dietetics. 2022. Available at: https://medlineplus.gov/ency/patientinstructions/000110.htm. Accessed Jun 20, 2022.

35. Pitt CE. Cutting Through the Paleo Hype: The Evidence for the Paleolithic Diet. Am Fam Physician 2016;45(1):35–8.

36. Harvard T. H. Chan School of Public Health. The Nutrition Source. Diet Review: Paleo Diet for Weight Loss. (n.d.) Available at: https://www.hsph.harvard.edu/nutritionsource/healthy-weight/diet-reviews/paleo-diet/. Accessed Jun 20, 2022.

37. Ghaedi E, Mohammadi M, Mohammadi H, et al. Effects of a paleolithic diet on cardiovascular disease risk factors: a systematic review and meta-analysis of randomized controlled trials. Adv Nutr 2019;10:634–46.

38. Martesson A, Stomby A, Tellstrom, et al. Using a paleo ratio to address adherence to paleolithic dietary recommendations in a randomized controlled trial of individuals with type 2 diabetes. Nutrients 2021;13:969.

39. Jamka M, Kulczynski B, Juruc A, et al. The effect of the paleolithic diet vs healthy diets on glucose and insulin homeostasis: a systematic review and meta-analysis of randomized controlled trials. J Clin Med 2020;9:296.

40. Welton S, Minty R, O'Driscoll T, et al. Intermittent fasting and weight loss: systematic review. Can Fam Physician 2020;66:117–25.

41. Patikom C, Roubal K, Veettil S, et al. Intermittent fasting and obesity-related health outcomes. an umbrella review of meta-analyses of randomized clinical trials. JAMA Netw Open 2021;4(12):e2139558.

42. What is intermittent fasting? Healthy lifestyle, nutrition and healthy eating. Mundi, Manpreet: Mayo Clinic; 2020.

43. Intermittent Fasting: What is it, and How Does it Work? Food and Nutrition. Johns Hopkins Medicine. (n.d.) Available at: https://www.hopkinsmedicine.org/health/wellness-and-prevention/intermittent-fasting-what-is-it-and-how-does-it-work. Accessed Jun 20, 2022.

44. Distribution of Diets Followed by Consumers in 2018 and 2019. 2022. Statista. • Consumer diet share U.S. Statista 2019. Available at: https://www.statista.com/statistics/993725/consumer-diet-share-us/. Accessed February 2022.

Nutrition and Cardiovascular Disease: An Update for Clinicians

Erin L. Sherer, EdD, PA-C, RD[a],*, Ahmad Hakemi, MD[b],
Andrew Lundahl, PharmD[d], Teresa L. Armstead, MA, BS[c],
Mishaal Malik, BS[e], Tyler M. Simmons, BS[f]

KEYWORDS

- Cardiovascular disease • Nutrition • Heart healthy • Dietary patterns
- American Heart Association • Dietary guidelines for Americans
- Dietary approaches to stop hypertension • Registered dietitian

KEY POINTS

- There are many modifiable risk factors for developing cardiovascular disease, including poor diet. Research indicates that improving nutritional status at an early age can reduce risk of cardiovascular disease development.
- Providing evidence-based nutrition guidance to patients can be confusing for clinicians owing to research limitations, media focus on controversial topics, and private sector influence.
- Past dietary guidelines focused on specific nutrients in the diet; however, current guidance suggests that healthy eating patterns beginning at birth may support cardiovascular health throughout life.
- Multiple healthy eating patterns can be adapted to individual preferences; those patterns with the most evidence for cardiovascular disease prevention include the Dietary Guidelines for Americans, the Mediterranean Diet, the Vegetarian Eating Pattern, and the Dietary Approaches to Stop Hypertension Diet.
- Research on improved cardiovascular nutrition is ongoing. Clinicians should understand that dietary guidelines are frequently revised according to emerging evidence.

INTRODUCTION

Cardiovascular disease (CVD) is a leading worldwide cause of disease and death.[1,2] Poor diet is one of the major risk factors for CVD, with estimates indicating that nearly

[a] Emergency Department, Columbia University Irving Medical Center, 622 West 168th Street, New York, NY 10032, USA; [b] Central Michigan University Physician Assistant Program, 1280 East Campus Drive, HPB Mailstop 2068, Mount Pleasant, MI 48859, USA; [c] Central Michigan University Physician Assistant Program, 1280 East Campus Drive, HPB 2076, Mount Pleasant, MI 48859, USA; [d] Mission Pharmacy, 926 Mission Street, Mount Pleasant, MI 48858, USA; [e] Central Michigan University, 1280 East Campus Drive, Mount Pleasant, MI 48859, USA; [f] Central Michigan University, 1280 East Campus Drive, HPB 1212, Mount Pleasant, MI 48859, USA
* Corresponding author.
E-mail address: els2183@tc.columbia.edu

Physician Assist Clin 7 (2022) 629–642
https://doi.org/10.1016/j.cpha.2022.05.003
physicianassistant.theclinics.com

80% of CVD deaths are attributed to this modifiable risk factor.[3–5] The Western diet—which is characterized by higher intakes of red meats, high-fat dairy products, and refined grains than elsewhere in the world—contributes to CVD and obesity.[6] Epidemiologic studies demonstrate a lower risk of CVD events associated with healthy diets in patients without prior CVD.[7] For these reasons, a heart-healthy diet has been recommended for the prevention and treatment of CVD.[8]

The idea of what constitutes a heart-healthy diet has evolved over the years. Previously, patients were urged to limit saturated fats, sodium, and cholesterol to specific amounts for the prevention and treatment of CVD.[9] However, current evidence instead supports improving diet quality through dietary components and patterns, rather than focusing on individual nutrients, foods, or even food groups.[9–12] Dietary components and patterns are simply the combinations of foods that people consume over time. Research indicates that, as a whole, certain foods work together to impact a person's health throughout their lifespan.[11] Current recommendations for heart-healthy dietary patterns encourage increased intakes of nutrient-dense foods, such as vegetables, fruits, whole grains, legumes, low-fat dairy, lean protein, and liquid oils in moderation.[11]

As nutritional science has advanced, it has changed. Certain nutrients, foods, and diets have received outsized focus and media attention, whereas others toil away in obscurity. This has led to confusion among clinicians and patients. This article aims to review and synthesize the most recent nutrition recommendations for reducing risk of CVD in an effort to provide clinicians with accurate information for enhancing patient education and care.

EVALUATING THE EVIDENCE

Research is a critical part of improving the understanding of how nutrition can impact CVD. Nutrition research includes many trials; however, not all studies provide useful information owing to a wide variety of issues, which include popular media tropes and fads that lodge themselves in the collective consciousness; confounding factors and the complex interplay of modern life; study design; and potential issues of influence within academia, industry, and elsewhere.

First, the "elephant in the room" must be addressed. On occasion, studies have found footing and are popularized in the media despite limited supporting evidence when it is clear that a story will capture audience attention. This has created confusion among clinicians, and even more consternation among the general population regarding what recommendations truly are for improving cardiovascular nutrition. Instead of seeking advertising revenue, registered dietitians (RDs) are nutrition experts who objectively evaluate and apply beneficial research findings to their work; RDs can and should be a valuable primary resource for clinicians and patients who are seeking research finding clarification or nutrition counseling.[13]

Another challenge to studying the impact of nutrition on long-term health is the wide array of confounding factors, as there is a complex interplay between nutrition, lifestyle behaviors, cultural beliefs, and socioeconomic factors that impact cardiovascular health.[9] Modifiable and nonmodifiable risk factors for CVD include age, family history, smoking, elevated blood pressure, abnormal cholesterol levels, elevated blood glucose levels, poor diet, and low levels of physical activity.[12,14–17] The natural history of disease progression also limits the availability of quality research. It can be difficult to determine the causal relationship between nutrition and major cardiovascular events when a disease process develops over a long period of time.

Study design also impacts research quality. Factors such as time constraints, associated costs, inability to blind participants, and an inability to obtain and maintain large sample sizes are all limiting factors for high-quality investigations.[18,19] Finally, research in this area has also been influenced by private sector funding.[20,21] This influence threatens the credibility of nutrition science, as it impacts nutrition policies and practices.[21] This may lead to a distrust of nutrition guidance by medical professionals and the public.[21]

CURRENT DIETARY GUIDELINES FOR PREVENTING CARDIOVASCULAR DISEASE

Many dietary guidelines were created with the prevention of CVD as a primary aim. Governmental agencies that include the US Department of Agriculture (USDA) and the US Department of Health and Human Services (HHS), and scientific societies that include the American Heart Association (AHA), the American College of Cardiology (ACC), and the World Health Organization (WHO) have all developed guidelines for reducing CVD risk through the promotion of healthy diet and lifestyle habits.[11,12,22] Clinicians giving advice or treatment in this area should have a basic understanding of the characteristics of these dietary recommendations as a foundation for understanding and assessing the validity of newer health claims and diets.

In general, evidence-based healthy dietary guidelines emphasize higher intakes of fruits, vegetables, whole grains, and legumes. The Dietary Guidelines for Americans (DGA), which are jointly updated every 5 years by the USDA and the HHS, focus on creating healthy dietary patterns by stages of life from birth through older adulthood.[11] The combined AHA and ACC recommendations, last revised in 2021, shifted the focus from nutrient-based to food-based, placing greater importance on healthy eating throughout one's life.[12] The latest WHO recommendations encourage a diversified, balanced, and healthy diet, placing emphasis on increased fruit and vegetable intake, and lower fat, sugar, and sodium intake (**Fig. 1**).[22]

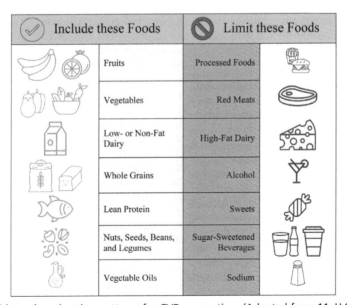

⊘ Include these Foods	🚫 Limit these Foods
Fruits	Processed Foods
Vegetables	Red Meats
Low- or Non-Fat Dairy	High-Fat Dairy
Whole Grains	Alcohol
Lean Protein	Sweets
Nuts, Seeds, Beans, and Legumes	Sugar-Sweetened Beverages
Vegetable Oils	Sodium

Fig. 1. Evidence-based eating patterns for CVD prevention. (Adapted from 11. U.S. Department of Agriculture and U.S. Department of Health and Human Services. Dietary Guidelines for Americans, 2020-2025. 9th Edition; and 12. Lichtenstein AH, Appel LJ, Vadiveloo M, et al. 2021 Dietary Guidance to Improve Cardiovascular Health: A Scientific Statement From the American Heart Association. *Circulation.* 2021;144(23)e472-487; and 22. Healthy Diet: World Health Organization. WHO.int. Published 2019. Accessed November 9, 2021.)

Within these guidelines, certain dietary patterns have been shown to prevent or improve CVD. Contemporary research has demonstrated that healthier diets and lifestyles, when compared with the conventional Western diet, are associated with fewer serum proinflammatory cytokines (namely C-reactive protein, interleukin-1 [IL-1], IL-6, IL-8, IL-18, and tumor necrosis factor-α), more anti-inflammatory cytokines, and ultimately, less atherosclerosis and CVD.[23,24] Accordingly, several dietary patterns have emerged as the most evidence-based recommendations when attempting to lower the risk of negative outcomes and mortality owing to CVD: the Healthy US Style Diet (HUSD), the Mediterranean Diet (MeD), the Vegetarian Eating Pattern (VD), and the Dietary Approaches to Stop Hypertension (DASH) diet.[11,25]

In December 2020, the USDA and HHS released the 9th edition of the DGA, which includes 3 different eating patterns: the HUSD, the MeD, and the VD. The DGA eating patterns promote 4 key principles of a healthy diet.[11] First, the 2020 to 2025 DGA encourages healthy eating at every life stage, starting with a recommendation for human breast milk for no less than the first year, and iron-fortified infant formula when breast milk is unattainable. Vitamin D supplementation soon after birth is also recommended for at least the first 6 months of life. Beyond 6 months, nutrient-dense and potentially allergenic foods are recommended along with foods rich in iron and zinc. Second, the DGA emphasizes the customizability of diets to cultures and budgets, highlighting the necessity for practicality. Third, the DGA endorses nutrient-dense and low-calorie foods, such as dark green, red, and orange vegetables, starchy vegetables, and beans, peas, and lentils. In particular, cruciferous vegetables (ie, broccoli, brussels sprouts, and cauliflower) have been shown to possess anti-inflammatory effects.[26,27] Fruits, whole grains, and fat-free or low-fat dairy, such as yogurt, milk, and cheese, are suggested. The DGA recommends nutritious proteins, which include lean meats, poultry, eggs, seafood, nuts, seeds, and soy products. When used sparingly, vegetable and olive oils are preferred as well as those found naturally in foods (ie, seafood and nuts). Less than 10% added sugars and saturated fats and fewer than 2300 mg of sodium are suggested. Alcoholic beverages are to be limited to 2 drinks or less a day for men and 1 drink or less for women. These guidelines closely resemble the DASH diet, which puts particular emphasis on lowering blood pressure, low-density lipoprotein cholesterol (LDL-C) levels, and limiting sodium intake to less than 1500 mg daily to minimize CVD risk in hypertensive individuals.[25]

The MeD, the eponymous eating pattern of those that live along the Mediterranean Sea, specifically in Spain, Italy, and Greece, emphasizes eating fruits, more healthy fats, and oils (like those in seafood and nuts) and less dairy than the HUSD provides for.[11] Numerous recent studies have confirmed the MeD's benefits in CVD and mortality reduction and improvements in metabolic disorders.[28,29] The Prevención con Dieta Mediterránea (PREDIMED) study was a multicenter, randomized, primary prevention trial aimed at evaluating the long-term effects of the MeD on CVD incidence.[30] PREDIMED involved more than 7000 Spanish men and women with high-risk CVD or type 2 diabetes mellitus (T2DM) and found that, when either placed on the MeD with oil or nuts and without any dietary fat or calorie restriction or advised to lower dietary fat, participants lowered their risk of negative cardiac events and T2DM by 30% and 52%, respectively.[30] PREDIMED was especially impactful, as it demonstrated that low-fat diets are not necessary to reduce heart disease risk. In fact, PREDIMED subjects had a total fat intake of 39% to 42% of total daily calories, largely from fish and nuts, which is significantly higher than the 20% to 35% recommendation in the DGA.

Furthermore, another 2018 study published in the *Journal of the American Medical Association* that analyzed 26,000 women on an MeD found a 25% reduced risk of CVD over 12 years.[31] The decreased risk was attributed to lower inflammation, lower blood sugar, and lower body mass index numbers.[31] Likewise, Shikany and colleagues[32,33] demonstrated that the MeD reduced coronary heart disease and sudden cardiac death in a diverse population compared with the Western and the "Southern" diet, characterized by added fats, fried food, eggs, organ and processed meats, and sugar-sweetened beverages in the REGARDS (Reasons for Geographic and Racial Differences in Stroke) trial.

The VD and variations on that theme have piqued Western interest in recent years but have also courted controversy regarding their advantages when compared with less-restrictive diet patterns. Current research supports the conclusion that there is a benefit from plant-based diets over the conventional Western diet in terms of weight status, glucose, cholesterol, and inflammation.[34,35] However, follow-up data regarding the benefits of plant-based diets beyond 1 year are scarce, which limits its reliability, as long-term success in a diet attenuates between 2 and 5 years.[36]

Although there is a great deal of focus on the type of diet pattern, there is strong evidence suggesting that general consumption of healthier foods and those higher in dietary quality provide cardiovascular benefits. The STABILITY (Stabilization of Atherosclerotic Plaque by Initiation of Darapladib Therapy) study evaluated the relationship between diet patterns and the incidence of major adverse cardiovascular events in high-risk patients with stable coronary artery disease.[37] The study of 15,482 patients from 39 countries found that it was more valuable for secondary prevention of coronary artery disease to consume healthy foods than it is to avoid less healthy foods found in Western diets.[37] Similarly, a prospective assessment of the TRANSCEND (Telmisartan Randomized Assessment Study in Angiotensin-Converting Enzyme Inhibitor (ACEI) Intolerant Subjects with Cardiovascular Disease) investigation and the ONTARGET (Ongoing Telmisartan Alone and in Combination with Ramipril Global EndPoint Trial) suggested that higher-quality diets are associated with lower risk for CVD events in older men and women with T2DM or CVD.[41] The evaluation suggested higher-quality diets in this patient population led to risk reductions for cardiovascular death, stroke, and myocardial infarction of 35%, 19%, and 14%, respectively.[38]

In summary, the current dietary guidelines emphasize improving overall nutrient quality and dietary patterns throughout one's life rather than focusing on specific foods or nutrients that appear in the diet. Given the research available, there is strong scientific support for recommending the 3 dietary patterns included in the DGA (Healthy US Style Diet, the Mediterranean Diet, the Vegetarian Eating Pattern) and the DASH diet for risk reduction and improvement in CVD risk factors.[10,11,25] Using these recommendations as a guide supports an eating pattern with underlying nutrient targets low in fats (saturated and trans); cholesterol; sodium; added sugars; and refined grains (**Table 1**).

SPECIFIC NUTRIENTS IMPORTANT IN CARDIOVASCULAR HEALTH
Fats

Dietary fat has probably received the most research and media attention over the years, likely because of the impact that saturated fat has on cholesterol levels.[39] There are different types of fats based on chemical composition that include trans, saturated, monounsaturated, and polyunsaturated. The 2 most harmful fats related to CVD are trans fats and saturated fats.[40] Trans fats develop through the process of hydrogenation, which turns liquid fats into solids, largely to prevent them from becoming rancid.[39] Saturated fats, found naturally in foods, increase blood levels of total cholesterol and LDL-C by decreasing hepatic LDL-C receptor synthesis, which in turn

Table 1
Recommended daily food portions of selected dietary patterns

	AHA/ACC[12] (for Adults)	DGA: Healthy US-Style[11] (Based on 2000 Calories for Ages 2 and Older)	DGA: Healthy Mediterranean-Style[11] (Based on 2000 Calories for Ages 2 and Older)	DGA: Healthy Vegetarian[11] (Based on 2000 Calories for Ages 2 and Older)	WHO Healthy Diet[22] (for Adults)
Vegetables	Eat plenty every day	2.5 cups per day	2.5 cups per day	2.5 cups per day	2.5 cups per day
Fruits	Eat plenty every day	2 cups per day	2 cups per day	2 cups per day	2 cups per day
Grains	Choose mostly whole grains instead of refined grains	6 ounces per day	6 ounces per day	6.5 ounces per day	180 g per day
Low-fat or nonfat dairy	Choose low-fat or nonfat instead of full fat	3 cups per day	2 cups per day	3 cups per day	Not included
Protein	Choose healthy sources	5.5 ounces per day	6.5 ounces per day	3.5 ounces per day	160 g
Oils	Choose liquid plant, rather than tropical, animal fats, and partially hydrogenated	27 g per day	27 g per day	27 g per day	Limit fat intake to <30% of daily energy intake
Limit on calories from foods from other sources	Minimize intake of beverages and foods with added sugars	240 calories per day	240 calories per day	250 calories per day	12 teaspoons per day (or 50 g)
Nuts, seeds, dry beans, and peas	Choose mostly plant-based protein sources	1.5 cups beans, peas, and lentils; 5 ounces nuts and seeds per week (included in vegetable and protein allotment)	1.5 cups beans, peas, and lentils; 5 ounces nuts and seeds per week (included in vegetable and protein allotment)	3 cups beans, peas, and lentils; 7 ounces nuts and seeds per week (included in vegetable and protein allotment)	(Included in protein allotment)
Alcohol	Limit intake	≤2 drinks per day for men and ≤1 drink per day for women	≤2 drinks per day for men and ≤1 drink per day for women	≤2 drinks per day for men and ≤1 drink per day for women	

reduces the removal of LDL-C from the circulation.[39] Trans fats are largely found in processed foods, such as margarine and baked goods, whereas saturated fats are found in red meats, full-fat dairy products, and oils produced from palm and coconut plants.[39] Evidence suggests that reducing dietary saturated fat and trans fat can decrease the risk of CVD.[38,39,40]

Unsaturated fats may occur in the form of polyunsaturated fatty acids (PUFAs) and monounsaturated fatty acids (MUFAs).[39] PUFAs are derived from nuts, seeds, avocados, and safflower oils, whereas sources of MUFAs include fish, olive oil, and nuts.[39] Omega-3 and omega-6 fatty acids are types of PUFAs that are essential in the diet.[39] Unsaturated fats are healthier than saturated and trans fats, as they do not impact cholesterol.[39] Knowing the difference between healthy and unhealthy fats is important and can assist in making better dietary choices.

Historically, low-fat diets have been recommended to prevent CVD; however, research has shown that diets with a moderate fat level (around 30%–35% of energy as fat, typical of the MeD) reduce CVD risk and may have increased adherence.[42] Saturated and trans fats should be limited and replaced with healthier fat sources, such as PUFAs and MUFAs.[40] The DGA and WHO recommend reducing saturated fats to less than 10% of total energy intake.[11,22] In 2015, the Food and Drug Administration withdrew trans fats from the Generally Recognized as Safe list.[38] This change has led to reductions of trans fat in the food supply and in food intake within the population.[38]

Cholesterol

Cholesterol is created in the body by the liver and naturally circulates through the body, but it can also be introduced into the body through food sources. Too much serum cholesterol can cause the waxy substance to slowly adhere to and build up in the inner walls of the arteries (atherosclerosis), which in turn may lead to CVD and an increased risk of a major cardiac event.[43] Two types of lipoproteins carry cholesterol to and from cells: LDL-C and high-density lipoprotein cholesterol (HDL-C). The "bad" cholesterol (LDL-C) contributes to atherosclerosis, whereas the "good" cholesterol (HDL-C) helps reduce atherosclerosis by transporting LDL-C away from the arteries and back to the liver for breakdown.[43]

Although saturated and trans fats have the biggest impact on blood cholesterol concentrations, cholesterol in foods also increases blood cholesterol concentrations.[9,44] Dietary guidelines historically recommended limiting dietary cholesterol intake to less than 300 mg per day, although more recent guidelines do not provide a specific numerical limit.[12] The 2020 to 2025 DGA recommends that "*trans* fat and dietary cholesterol consumption be as low as possible without compromising the nutritional adequacy of the diet."[11] This change was first noted in the 2015 to 2020 DGA owing to a lack of evidence for an appreciable relationship between dietary and serum cholesterol levels and is consistent with the current recommendations from the AHA.[12,44] The debate regarding whether dietary cholesterol should be limited occurs because dietary cholesterol increases serum lipids nonlinearly, and the effect of dietary cholesterol depends on the baseline lipid levels.[44]

Sodium

Sodium is an essential nutrient in our diets most commonly found in the form of salt (sodium chloride). Sodium is used in many foods as a preservative and is also frequently added to enhance flavor to taste. Unfortunately, a high dietary intake of sodium has been found to be a risk factor for CVD, and there is a direct positive correlation between salt intake and blood pressure.[12,45] Randomized trials indicate that lowering sodium intake reduces blood pressure levels, thereby lowering risk of CVD.[46] However, it is important to note that lowering sodium intake below the recommended levels does not offer much benefit.[46]

Maintaining a normal blood pressure is an important step in preventing CVD; consuming a low sodium diet is one approach to achieving this. The DASH trial demonstrated that consuming a diet high in fruits, vegetables, low-fat dairy products, and low in saturated fat and cholesterol thereby lowered both systolic blood pressure and diastolic blood pressure.[25] Follow-up trials also showed there was a stepwise reduction in blood pressure depending on the level of sodium in the diet and that reducing sodium intake combined with the DASH diet also lowered blood pressure.[47,48]

Limiting sodium intake can be challenging because of its ubiquity, ease of encounter, and the difficulty of procuring acceptable alternatives. Sodium content is typically higher in processed foods and those prepared at restaurants.[11] The 2020 to 2025 DGA indicates the average daily sodium intake in the United States for those ages 1 and older is 3393 mg per day.[11] Although the AHA/ACC recommendations simply state, "choose and prepare foods with little or no salt," the DGA suggests a daily sodium intake limit for adults of less than 2300 mg per day.[11,12] Different strategies to reduce dietary sodium should be implemented, including cooking at home more often, reading nutrition labels to choose products containing sodium levels less than 140 mg per serving, and using spices and ingredients other than salt to add flavor to food.[11]

Potassium

Potassium is an important mineral the human body uses to regulate blood pressure. In addition to helping muscles contract, potassium regulates fluid and mineral balance in the cells and also limits the effect that salt has on blood pressure.[49] There is a well-documented inverse relationship between potassium intake and blood pressure.[46,50] The effects of potassium on blood pressure depend on the associated intake of salt (or lack thereof). For example, a high potassium intake lowers blood pressure when there is also a high sodium intake.[51] Several studies, including the previously discussed DASH trial, have concluded that cardiovascular damage and death accelerated by elevated blood pressure associated with high salt intake could be prevented by increased dietary potassium intake.[25,50,52] A meta-analysis of potassium intake and CVD revealed higher daily potassium intakes of 3500 mg to 4700 mg were associated with a reduction in blood pressure in hypertensive patients and a 24% lower risk of stroke.[52] There are currently no Recommended Dietary Allowance (RDA) levels for potassium; however, the National Academy of Medicine has established Adequate Intake (AI) for potassium. For women aged 19 and older, the AI is 2600 mg per day and for men agef 19 and older the AI is 3600 mg per day.[49]

Although potassium supplements are available, this mineral can easily be increased in the diet through food sources. Potassium-rich foods include most fruits and vegetables, dairy products, meat, poultry, fish, and nuts[49] (**Table 2**).

Added Sugar

Sugar from carbohydrate intake is vital, as it provides energy for the body.[53] Carbohydrates are broken down into glucose, and although glucose is not the main source of energy during aerobic metabolism, it still provides a major source of ATP for the myocardium.[54] Although glucose is an essential nutrient in maintaining homeostasis, the AHA attributes 8.8% of CVD events to abnormal blood glucose.[55] Chronic hyperglycemia, as seen in T2DM, causes damage and dysfunction to the heart and blood vessels.[55] The influence of excess glucose seen in diabetes has a devastating effect

Table 2
Quantitative nutrient-based recommendations and targets in selected dietary patterns

Dietary Pattern	Quantitative Nutrient-Based Recommendations	Underlying Nutrient-Based Targets Found Within Dietary Pattern
DASH Diet[25]	• Limit total fat to 27% of energy intake per day • Limit saturated fat to 6% of energy intake per day • Limit cholesterol to 150 mg per day • Limit sodium to 2300 mg per day (limit to 1500 mg per day if have risk factors) • Consume 4700 mg of potassium per day • Consume 500 mg of magnesium per day	• Specific targets provided
2020–2025 dietary guidelines for Americans[11]	• Limit saturated fat to <10% of total energy intake per day • Limit added sugars to <10% of total energy intake per day • Limit sodium intake to <2300 mg per day	• Saturated fat, sodium, and added sugar targets provided • Dietary patterns are limited in trans fat and cholesterol

on the microvasculature, the larger arteries, the heart, and the kidneys—so much so that diabetes has a coequal status with hypertension, tobacco smoking, and dyslipidemia as a major risk factor for CVD.[53] Given sufficient time to progress, diabetes will cause cardiac remodeling and atherosclerosis, which in turn may lead to coronary artery disease, myocardial infarction, or stroke.[55]

Evidence indicates that limiting the intake of added sugars and sugar-sweetened beverages is important for reducing the risk of developing T2DM, CVD, and excess weight gain.[12,39,56] Common types of added sugars include glucose, dextrose, sucrose, corn syrup, honey, maple syrup, and concentrated fruit juice.[12,39] On average, added sugars account for approximately 13% of total calories per day (or about 270 calories) in the US population.[11] Different organizations have varying opinions on how much added sugar is safe to consume without impacting future health.[56] The AHA offers a general recommendation that individuals minimize the intake of beverages and foods with added sugars, whereas the DGA indicates individuals should consume less than 10% of their calories per day from added sugars starting at age 2.[11,12] An easy way to reduce added sugar in the diet is to eliminate or limit sugar-sweetened beverages, as data indicate this is the highest source of added sugars in the American diet.[11]

Magnesium

Magnesium is another important nutrient for cardiovascular health. Higher levels of circulating magnesium are associated with lower risk of CVD.[57] This mineral fulfills numerous physiologic roles in the proper functioning of the cardiac muscle, including an important function in active ionic transport (Ca^{++} and K^+) across cardiac cell membranes, a process that is necessary for maintaining a normal sinus rhythm, nerve impulse conduction, and myocardial contraction.[58,59] Hypomagnesemia has numerous CVD complications, with the most ominous of all torsades de pointes and ventricular tachycardia.[60] Other deleterious effects of magnesium deficiency include supraventricular tachycardia, atrial fibrillation, hypertension, and increased risk of thrombotic events.[58,59]

Magnesium is monitored through routine serum levels, and it is of utmost importance that clinicians' thresholds for ordering serum magnesium be very low, as magnesium deficiency may be underdiagnosed.[59,61] The RDA for magnesium in adults is 420 mg.[59] Rich food sources of this nutrient include nuts, seeds, beans, green leafy vegetables, whole-wheat bread, and oatmeal.[59]

SUMMARY

Instead of focusing on single nutrients or foods, evidence suggests that providers should encourage an overall healthful dietary pattern throughout an individual's lifespan for CVD prevention. Although specific nutrients certainly do play roles in the development of CVD, research on isolated nutrients indicates that the development of CVD is multifactorial; therefore, focusing on one nutrient in the diet can be challenging, may not offer much benefit, and could distract from the importance of a holistic approach. Although some dietary guidelines continue to make nutrient-based recommendations, most dietary patterns are rooted in, and compliant with, evidence-based nutrient targets. This trend toward dietary pattern–based eating should make it easier for clinicians and patients to better understand the recommendations for cardiovascular nutrition.

CLINICS CARE POINTS

- Healthy dietary patterns should be encouraged starting at birth and continuing throughout the lifespan.
- Evidence-based dietary patterns that support prevention of cardiovascular disease include the following:
  - The Healthy US Style Diet (Dietary Guidelines for Americans 2020–2025)
  - The Mediterranean Diet
  - The Vegetarian Eating Pattern
  - The DASH Diet
- Patient education should emphasize consumption of healthy fats, reduction of excess cholesterol, sodium, and added sugars within the eating pattern.
- Clinicians should remember that making dietary changes is often challenging for patients, and there may be socioeconomic and cultural factors that can impede patients from adopting healthy lifestyle habits.
- Clinicians may wish to consider evaluating serum nutrient levels in patients on an individual basis to make further dietary recommendations.
- Reduction of other modifiable cardiovascular disease risk factors should also be encouraged, including maintenance of normal weight, adequate physical activity, control of cholesterol, blood pressure, and blood sugar as well as tobacco avoidance.[12]

DISCLOSURE

The authors have nothing to disclose.

REFERENCES

1. GBD 2013 Mortality and Causes of Death Collaborators. Global, regional, and national age–sex specific all-cause and cause-specific mortality for 240 causes of death, 1990–2013: a systematic analysis for the Global Burden of Disease Study 2013. Lancet 2015;385(9963):117–71.
2. Virani SS, Alonso A, Aparicio HJ, et al. Heart disease and stroke statistics—2021 Update: a report from the American Heart Association. Circulation 2021; 143:e254–743.
3. Murray CJ. The State of US Health, 1990-2010. JAMA 2013;310(6):591–608.
4. Stampfer MJ, Hu FB, Manson JE, et al. Primary prevention of coronary heart disease in women through diet and lifestyle. N Engl J Med 2000;343(1):16–22.
5. Yusuf S, Hawken S, Ôunpuu S, et al. Effect of potentially modifiable risk factors associated with myocardial infarction in 52 countries (the INTERHEART study): case-control study. Lancet 2004;364(9438):937–52.
6. Fung TT, Rimm EB, Spiegelman D, et al. Association between dietary patterns and plasma biomarkers of obesity and cardiovascular disease risk. Am J Clin Nutr 2001;73(1):61–7.
7. Knoops KT, de Groot LC, Kromhout D, et al. Mediterranean diet, lifestyle factors, and 10-year mortality in elderly European men and women: the HALE project. JAMA 2004;292:1433–9.
8. American Heart Association. The American Heart Association's diet and lifestyle recommendations. Heart.org. 2015. Available at: https://www.heart.org/en/healthy-living/healthy-eating/eat-smart/nutrition-basics/aha-diet-and-lifestyle-recommendations. Accessed January 21, 2022.
9. Freeman AM, Morris PB, Barnard N, et al. Trending cardiovascular nutrition controversies. J Am Coll Cardiol 2017;69(9):1172–87.
10. Shan Z, Li Y, Baden MY, et al. Association between healthy eating patterns and risk of cardiovascular disease. JAMA Intern Med 2020;180(8):1090.
11. U.S. Department of Agriculture and U.S. Department of Health and Human Services. Dietary guidelines for Americans, 2020-2025. DietaryGuidelines.gov. 9th edition 2020. Available at: https://www.dietaryguidelines.gov/sites/default/files/2020-12/Dietary_Guidelines_for_Americans_2020-2025.pdf. Accessed December 26, 2021.
12. Lichtenstein AH, Appel LJ, Vadiveloo M, et al. 2021 dietary guidance to improve cardiovascular health: a scientific statement from the American Heart Association. Circulation 2021;144(23):e472–87.
13. What is a Registered Dietitian Nutritionist? Eatrightpro.org. Available at: https://www.eatrightpro.org/about-us/what-is-an-rdn-and-dtr/what-is-a-registered-dietitian-nutritionist. Accessed January 22, 2022.
14. Stone NJ, Robinson JG, Lichtenstein AH, et al. 2013 ACC/AHA guideline on the treatment of blood cholesterol to reduce atherosclerotic cardiovascular risk in adults: a report of the American College of Cardiology/American Heart Association Task Force on Practice Guidelines. Circulation 2014;129(25 Suppl 2):S1–45.
15. Jacobson TA, Maki KC, Orringer CE, et al. National Lipid Association recommendations for patient-centered management of dyslipidemia: part 2. J Clin Lipidol 2015;9(6 Suppl):S1–122.e1.
16. Whelton PK, Carey RM, Aronow WS, et al. 2017 ACC/AHA/AAPA/ABC/ACPM/AGS/APhA/ASH/ASPC/NMA/PCNA guideline for the prevention, detection, evaluation, and management of high blood pressure in adults: a report of the American College of Cardiology/American Heart Association Task Force on Clinical

Practice Guidelines. Heart.org. 2017. Available at: http://hyper.ahajournals.org/content/hypertensionaha/early/2017/11/10/HYP.0000000000000065.full.pdf. Accessed October 19, 2021.

17. Eckel RH, Jakicic JM, Ard JD, et al. 2013 AHA/ACC guideline on lifestyle management to reduce cardiovascular risk: a report of the American College of Cardiology/American Heart Association Task Force on Practice Guidelines. Circulation 2014;129(25 Suppl 2):S76–99.

18. Maki KC, Slavin JL, Rains TM, et al. Limitations of observational evidence: implications for evidence-based dietary recommendations. Adv Nutr 2014;5:7–15.

19. Willett WC. Nutrition and chronic disease. Public Health Rev 1998;26:9–10.

20. Kearns CE, Schmidt LA, Glantz SA. Sugar industry and coronary heart disease research: a historical analysis of internal industry documents. JAMA Intern Med 2016;176:1680–5.

21. Nestle M. Corporate funding of food and nutrition research: science or marketing? JAMA Intern Med 2016;176(1):13–4.

22. Healthy diet: world health organization. WHO.int; 2019. Available at: https://apps.who.int/iris/bitstream/handle/10665/325828/EMROPUB_2019_en_23536.pdf. Accessed November 9, 2021.

23. Sijtsma FP, Meyer KA, Steffen LM, et al. Diet quality and markers of endothelial function: the CARDIA study. Nutr Metab Cardiovasc Dis 2014;24(6):632–8.

24. Piccand E, Vollenweider P, Guessous I, et al. Association between dietary intake and inflammatory markers: results from the CoLaus study. Public Health Nutr 2018;22(3):498–505.

25. Appel LJ, Moore TJ, Obarzanek E, et al, DASH Collaborative Research Group. A clinical trial of the effects of dietary patterns on blood pressure. N Engl J Med 1997;336:1117–24.

26. Jiang Y, Wu S-H, Shu X-O, et al. Cruciferous Vegetable intake is inversely correlated with circulating levels of proinflammatory markers in women. J Acad Nutr Diet 2014;114(5):700–8.e2.

27. Yagishita Y, Fahey JW, Dinkova-Kostova AT, et al. Broccoli or sulforaphane: is it the source or dose that matters? Molecules 2019;24(19):3593.

28. Viscogliosi G, Cipriani E, Liguori ML, et al. Mediterranean dietary pattern adherence: associations with prediabetes, metabolic syndrome, and related microinflammation. Metab Syndr Relat Disord 2013;11(3):210–6.

29. Grosso G, Marventano S, Yang J, et al. A comprehensive meta-analysis on evidence of Mediterranean diet and cardiovascular disease: Are individual components equal? Crit Rev Food 2015;57(15):3218–32.

30. Estruch R, Ros E, Salas-Salvadó J, et al. Primary prevention of cardiovascular disease with a Mediterranean diet. N Engl J Med 2013;368(14):1279–90.

31. Ahmad S, Moorthy MV, Demler OV, et al. Assessment of risk factors and biomarkers associated with risk of cardiovascular disease among women consuming a Mediterranean diet. JAMA Netw Open 2018;1(8):e185708.

32. Shikany JM, Safford MM, Soroka O, et al. Mediterranean diet score, dietary patterns, and risk of sudden cardiac death in the REGARDS study. J Am Heart Assoc 2021;10(13). https://doi.org/10.1161/jaha.120.019158.

33. Shikany JM, Safford MM, Newby PK, et al. Southern dietary pattern is associated with hazard of acute coronary heart disease in the reasons for geographic and racial differences in stroke (REGARDS) study. Circulation 2015;132(9):804–14.

34. Huang R-Y, Huang C-C, Hu FB, et al. Vegetarian diets and weight reduction: a meta-analysis of randomized controlled trials. J Gen Intern Med 2016;31(1):109–16.

35. Benatar JR, Stewart RAH. Cardiometabolic risk factors in vegans; A meta-analysis of observational studies. In: Chen O, editor. PLoS One 2018;13(12): e0209086.
36. Wing RR, Phelan S. Long-term weight loss maintenance. Am J Clin Nutr 2005; 82(1):222S225S.
37. Stewart RA, Wallentin L, Benatar J, et al. Dietary patterns and the risk of major adverse cardiovascular events in a global study of high-risk patients with stable coronary heart disease. Eur Heart J 2016;37(25):1993–2001.
38. Dehghan M, Mente A, Teo KK, et al. Relationship between healthy diet and risk of cardiovascular disease among patients on drug therapies for secondary prevention: a prospective cohort study of 31 546 high-risk individuals from 40 countries. Circulation 2012;126(23):2705–12.
39. Stanner S, Coe S, Frayn KN, et al. Cardiovascular Disease: Diet, Nutrition and Emerging Risk Factors. Wiley; 2019. https://doi.org/10.1002/9781118829875.
40. The facts on fats: 50 years of American Heart Association Dietary Fats Recommendations. Heart.org. 2015. Available at: https://www.heart.org/-/media/files/healthy-living/company-collaboration/inap/fats-white-paper-ucm_475005.pdf. Accessed October 12, 2021.
41. Sacks FM, Lichtenstein AH, Wu JH, et al. American Heart Association. Dietary fats and cardiovascular disease: a presidential advisory from the American Heart Association. Circulation 2017;136:e1–23.
42. Azadbakht L, Mirmiran P, Esmaillzadeh A, et al. Better dietary adherence and weight maintenance achieved by a long-term moderate-fat diet. Br J Nutr 2007;97(2):399–404. https://doi.org/10.1017/S0007114507328602.
43. American Heart Association. Control Your Cholesterol. Heart.org. 2017. Available at: https://www.heart.org/en/health-topics/cholesterol/about-cholesterol. Accessed December 22, 2021.
44. Bowen KJ, Sullivan VK, Kris-Etherton PM, et al. Nutrition and cardiovascular disease—an update. Curr Atheroscler Rep 2018;20(2). https://doi.org/10.1007/s11883-018-0704-3.
45. He FJ, MacGregor GA. Reducing population salt intake worldwide: From evidence to implementation. Prog Cardiovasc Dis 2010;52(5):363–82. https://doi.org/10.1016/j.pcad.2009.12.006.
46. Stallings VA, Harrison M, Oria M, editors. Dietary reference intakes for sodium and potassium. National Academies Press; 2019. https://doi.org/10.17226/25353.
47. Sacks FM, Svetkey LP, Vollmer WM, et al. DASH-Sodium Collaborative Research Group. Effects on blood pressure of reduced dietary sodium and the Dietary Approaches to Stop Hypertension (DASH) diet. N Engl J Med 2001;344:3–10.
48. Juraschek SP, Miller ER, Weaver CM, et al. Effects of sodium reduction and the DASH diet in relation to baseline blood pressure. J Am Coll Cardiol 2017; 70(23):2841–8.
49. What is potassium? Eatright.org. 2019. Available at: https://www.eatright.org/food/vitamins-and-supplements/types-of-vitamins-and-nutrients/what-is-potassium. Accessed January 2, 2022.
50. Kanbay M, Bayram Y, Solak Y, et al. Dietary potassium: a key mediator of the cardiovascular response to dietary sodium chloride. J Am Soc Hypertens 2013;7(5): 395–400.
51. Appel LJ, Brands MW, Daniels SR, et al. Dietary approaches to prevent and treat hypertension: a scientific statement from the American Heart Association. Hypertension 2006;47(2):296–308.

52. Aburto NJ, Hanson S, Gutierrez H, et al. Effect of increased potassium intake on cardiovascular risk factors and disease: systematic review and meta-analyses. BMJ 2013;346:f1378.
53. Diabetes mellitus: a major risk factor for cardiovascular disease. A joint editorial statement by the American Diabetes Association; The National Heart, Lung, and Blood Institute; The Juvenile Diabetes Foundation International; The National Institute of Diabetes and Digestive and Kidney Diseases; and The American Heart Association. Circulation 1999;100(10):1132–3.
54. Dods RF. Understanding diabetes. John Wiley & Sons, Inc.; 2013. https://doi.org/10.1002/9781118530665.
55. Peplow P, Adams J, Young T. Cardiovascular and metabolic disease: scientific discoveries and new therapies. Royal Society of Chemistry; 2015.
56. Rippe JM, Angelopoulos TJ. Fructose-containing sugars and cardiovascular disease. Adv Nutr 2015;6(4):430–9.
57. Rosique-Esteban N, Guasch-Ferré M, Hernández-Alonso P, et al. Dietary magnesium and cardiovascular disease: A review with emphasis in epidemiological studies. Nutrients 2018;10(2):168.
58. Jahnen-Dechent W, Ketteler M. Magnesium basics. Clin Kidney J 2012;5(Suppl 1):i3–14.
59. National Institutes of Health. Office of Dietary Supplements - Magnesium. Nih.gov. 2016. Available at: https://ods.od.nih.gov/factsheets/Magnesium-HealthProfessional/. Accessed October 12, 2021.
60. Mackay JD, Bladon PT. Hypomagnesaemia due to proton-pump inhibitor therapy: a clinical case series. QJM 2010;103(6):387–95.
61. DiNicolantonio JJ, O'Keefe JH, Wilson W. Subclinical magnesium deficiency: a principal driver of cardiovascular disease and a public health crisis. Open Heart 2018;5(1):e000668 [published correction appears in Open Heart. 2018 Apr 5;5(1):e000668corr1].

Medical Nutrition Therapy for Glycemic Control

Lorraine Laccetti Mongiello, DrPH, RDN, CDE

KEYWORDS

- Medical nutrition therapy • Glycemic control • Time in range
- Diabetes self-management education and support

KEY POINTS

- An appropriate diet is the cornerstone of diabetes management.
- There is no single specific "diet" recommended for diabetes.
- Nutrition guidance must be individualized based on numerous factors and glycemic goals.
- Carbohydrates have the greatest impact on postprandial blood glucose.
- All those using insulin should be offered education on how to match insulin to carbohydrate intake to increase meal flexibility and improve outcomes.

INTRODUCTION

In the United States, more than 37.3 million (11.3%) adults are living with diabetes and an additional 96 million (38.0%) with prediabetes.[1] Of these, 8.5 million have not yet been diagnosed.[2] As up to 70% of people with prediabetes are likely to develop type 2 diabetes during their lifetimes,[3] the prevalence of diabetes in the United States is projected to increase to 100 million people by 2050.[4]

Both the prevalence of diabetes and the risk of developing the disease vary widely with race and ethnicity. This difference in prevalence reflects differences in both the susceptibility to the disease as well as to the social determinates of health.[5] Black and Hispanic populations are approximately twice as likely to develop diabetes as whites, but disparities are most prominent among South Asians living in the United States. They have the highest age-adjusted burden of diabetes (23%), and South Asians are more than 3 times as likely to develop diabetes as their white counterparts.[6,7] Notably, the onset of diabetes in Asians occurs at a lower body mass index (BMI) than in other groups,[6] requiring the use of ethnic-specific BMI cutoff points for assessing diabetes risk.[8]

Because people with diabetes are at increased risk for numerous complications, diabetes has become the most expensive chronic disease in this country. At a cost

Clinical Nutrition & Interdisciplinary Health Sciences, New York Institute of Technology, Old Westbury, NY 11568-8000, USA
E-mail address: lmongiel@NYIT.edu

Physician Assist Clin 7 (2022) 643–654
https://doi.org/10.1016/j.cpha.2022.05.005
2405-7991/22/© 2022 Elsevier Inc. All rights reserved.

of $327 billion annually,[9] it is not only an individual hardship but a substantial economic and public health burden as well.

Effective blood glucose management is the key to reducing this burden, and appropriate food choices are key to optimal glycemia. There are several important measures of glycemic control. Hemoglobin A1C (A1C) is currently the primary measure to guide diabetes management. Although it does not document the daily highs and lows, it is still a useful indicator of overall control and a predictor of complications.[10,11] Postprandial blood glucose is an important indicator used to assess the impact of diet. For those using continuous glucose monitors, time-in-range (TIR) is emerging as a very valuable indicator of glycemia. The general consensus is that most people with diabetes should aim for a TIR, between 70 and 180 mg/dL, at least 70% of the time (roughly 17 out of 24 hours).[12] The incorporation of TIR metrics into clinical practice is growing and evolving, and remote access to these data can be advantageous for telemedicine.[13]

The American Association of Clinical Endocrinologists (AACE)[14] and the American Diabetes Association (ADA)[13] each provide guidelines for setting glycemic targets (**Box 1**). The ADA guidelines tend to be used by general practitioners, whereas the AACE guidelines are more commonly followed by endocrinologists because of the more aggressive targets. Both groups recommend the need for individualization based on factors such as life expectancy, social support, access to care, and patient motivation.[13,14]

This review discusses the fundamental role of medical nutrition therapy (MNT) in achieving these targets for both type 1 and type 2 diabetes. Maintaining glycemic control can reduce the risk of eye disease, kidney disease, and nerve disease by 40%.[10] Diet and lifestyle changes that improve blood pressure can reduce the risk of heart disease and stroke by 33% to 50%,[15] and improved cholesterol levels can reduce cardiovascular complications by 20% to 50%.[16]

MEDICAL NUTRITION THERAPY

MNT is defined as the treatment of a disease or condition through the modification of nutrients or whole-food intake.[17] It is the legal definition of nutrition counseling that is provided by a registered dietitian/nutritionist (RDN).[18]

The RDN's specialized academic preparation, training, and skills make them the preferred member of the interprofessional diabetes care team to provide nutrition assessment, nutrition diagnosis, diet education, food-related counseling, and monitoring with ongoing follow-up to support long-term lifestyle changes, evaluate outcomes of diet changes, and modify interventions as needed.[17,19] For diabetes management, a dietitian with an advanced certification (Certified Diabetes Educator or Board Certified-Advanced Diabetes Management) is ideal but not required.[17]

Strong evidence supports the fact that effectiveness of MNT provided by RDNs for A1C decreases up to 2.0% in type 2 diabetes and up to 1.9% in type 1 diabetes.[20] This 2017 systematic review also reported that A1C reductions from MNT can be similar to or

Box 1 Glycemic targets	
AACE[14]	**ADA[13]**
A1C ≤6.5% (less stringent for "less healthy")	A1C <7% (lower levels may be appropriate)
FBS 70–110 mg/dL	FBS 80–130 mg/dL
2 h after meals <140 mg/dL	Peak postprandial <180 mg/dL
Abbreviation: FBS, fasting blood sugar.	

greater than what is expected with current pharmacologic treatments.[20] In addition, the cost-effectiveness of MNT for glycemic control has been strongly demonstrated; it is a covered Medicare benefit for both those with diabetes and those with prediabetes and is typically reimbursed by most other payers.[18,21,22] Therefore, the American Academy of Nutrition and Dietetics and the ADA, and others, recommend that providers refer people with diabetes for nutrition counseling at diagnosis and as needed though the lifespan when there is a change in circumstance or if not achieving targets.[19]

Although the RDN is the primary provider of nutrition counseling and education, it is essential that all members of the health care team are aware of the goals of MNT (**Box 2**) and have the knowledge to help their patients achieve them. It is of vital importance that health care providers are equipped to counter the barrage of deceptive, manipulative, incomplete, inaccurate, or downright dangerous nutrition information that their patients receive from social media.[23,24] An analysis of millions of social media posts found that false stories were 70% more likely to be shared than true stories,[25] and most of the health-diet related tweets in 2018 to 2019 originated primarily from 10 influential accounts, including South Beach Diet, PETA, NetMeds (an offshore pharmaceutical company), and Donald Trump.[24] In 2021, the surgeon general proclaimed that this spread of misinformation through social media has become an "urgent threat to public health."[26]

Being diagnosed with diabetes is a physical, emotional, mental, and financial drain. Conflicting food and nutrition advice can leave patients and their families feeling even more overwhelmed, confused, and distressed. They simply want to know what to eat.

MACRONUTRIENTS

Unfortunately, there is no simple answer to the question "what can I eat." Although it would certainly make dietary instruction easier, the ideal percentage of calories from carbohydrate, protein, and fat for people with diabetes is simply not known.[27] Nor is it likely that there is a specific "diabetic diet" due to the wide range of differences among those with the disease. In addition to the multifactorial cause of the disease and numerous comorbidities, the dietitian needs to consider cultural backgrounds, food preferences, budget, and access to food. Therefore, macronutrient distribution and energy requirements must be individualized following an assessment of current eating patterns, patient preferences, and treatment goals.[17]

Box 2
Goals of nutrition therapy for adults with diabetes; American Diabetes Association Standards of Care 2022[19]

1. To promote and support healthful eating patterns, emphasizing a variety of nutrient-dense foods in appropriate portion sizes, to improve overall health and
   - achieve and maintain body weight goals
   - attain individualized glycemic, blood pressure, and lipid goals
   - delay or prevent the complications of diabetes

2. To address individual nutrition needs based on personal and cultural preferences, health literacy and numeracy, access to healthful foods, willingness and ability to make behavioral changes, and existing barriers to change

3. To maintain the pleasure of eating by providing nonjudgmental messages about food choices while limiting food choices only when indicated by scientific evidence

4. To provide an individual with diabetes the practical tools for developing healthy eating patterns rather than focusing on individual macronutrients, micronutrients, or single foods

Carbohydrates are the most quickly used source of energy and the primary dietary determinate of postprandial blood glucose. The amount of carbohydrate intake required for optimal health for people, with or without diabetes, is unknown. Although there is a recommended dietary allowance for carbohydrate of 130 g/d, it can be fulfilled by the body's metabolic processes such as gluconeogenesis and not necessarily dependent on intake.[28] The ADA recommendations regarding carbohydrates are found in **Box 3**.

Low-carbohydrate diets ($\leq$40%–45% of calories from carbohydrate) are among the most studied and common eating patterns for type 2 diabetes. They have been shown to reduce A1C and the need for oral hypoglycemic agents.[29,30] Reducing overall carbohydrate intake for individuals with diabetes may be applied in a variety of eating patterns that meet individual needs and preferences such as the Mediterranean or DASH diets.[17]

An effective meal-planning method used in diabetes management to help optimize blood glucose control is carbohydrate counting.[31] It can be used with or without the use of insulin therapy. At its most basic level it involves limiting the number of grams of carbohydrate in a meal based on an individual's postprandial glucose response. This method includes an assessment of current dietary intake followed by individualized guidance on self-monitoring of both carbohydrate intake, medications, and postprandial blood glucose. Based on this assessment a carbohydrate "allowance" is determined for each meal. It is important to note that although all sources of carbohydrates (starches, fruits, milk, and sweets) are included in this method, patients should be encouraged to choose primarily from fruit, vegetables, whole grains, beans, and low-fat or nonfat milk and limit added sugars, refined grains, and processed foods. Sugar-sweetened beverages, fruit juice, sports drinks, and energy drinks are best avoided altogether.

Advanced carbohydrate counting training should be offered to all individuals with type 1 or type 2 diabetes taking mealtime insulin.[19] Intensive and ongoing education is required to teach patients how to match insulin dosing with carbohydrate intake. For detailed guidance in teaching both basic and advanced carbohydrate counting, refer to the *Carbohydrate Primer for Primary Care Providers* article in this issue.

There is not one specific definition of a low carbohydrate diet, and the Food and Drug Administration (FDA) does not allow "low carb" (nor should it) on labels.

It is known that consumers often misinterpret labels and cannot accurately estimate the quantities they describe.[32] Unfamiliar terms on labels such as "net carbs" (which has no standard meaning), dietetic, sugar alcohols, glycemic index, glycemic load,

---

Box 3
Carbohydrates: key recommendations—American Diabetes Association Standards of Care 2022[19]

1. Nutrient-dense carbohydrate sources that are high in fiber (at least 14 g fiber per 1000 kcal), minimally processed, and without added sugar should be emphasized, such as nonstarchy vegetables, fruits, whole grains, and low-fat dairy products.

2. People with diabetes are advised to replace sugar-sweetened beverages (including fruit juices) with water as much as possible to control glycemia and weight and reduce their risk for cardiovascular disease and fatty liver disease.

3. When using a flexible insulin therapy program, education on the glycemic impact of carbohydrate should be provided to optimize mealtime insulin dosing.

4. When using fixed insulin doses, individuals should be provided education about maintaining a consistent pattern of carbohydrate intake with respect to time and amount.

and artificially sweetened add to the confusion. So, when providing guidance for people with diabetes, if a carbohydrate intake is to be recommended, it should be given in number of grams rather than percentages, as determining the percentage of calories from carbohydrate is daunting for patients, whereas grams are clearly indicated on all Nutrition Facts Labels.

The glycemic index (GI) is a measure of the relative area under the curve of a 50-g carbohydrate compared with a 50-g standard food such as bread or glucose.[33] Foods with a low GI are typically rich in fiber, protein, and/or fat and may cause a slower increase in blood glucose and should be encouraged.[20] However, a food's GI ranking does not take into account how much is consumed and is valid only when a food is consumed on an empty stomach without any other food or beverage.[33] Glycemic load (GL) corrects for a potentially misleading GI by multiplying the carbohydrate content of the portion by the food's GI, then that number is divided by 100.[33] Calculating the GI and GL is clearly complicated and offers little to improve glycemic control. For these reasons is generally not recommended as a meal-planning method.[20,31]

There are numerous FDA-approved nonnutritive (artificial) sweeteners containing very few or no calories. For those who are accustomed to regularly consuming sugar-sweetened products, these sweeteners can be an acceptable substitute for carbohydrate, as they do not have a significant effect on postprandial glycemia and they can reduce overall calorie and carbohydrate intake.[17]

Protein research is inconclusive regarding the ideal amount for glycemic management or minimizing cardiovascular disease (CVD) risk. There is no evidence that people with diabetes require either more or less of the recommended daily allowance (0.8 g/kg); this includes those with diabetic kidney disease.[34] However, successful management of type 2 diabetes typically requires meal plans with higher levels of protein required to replace carbohydrates; this has the added potential benefit of increased satiety.[35] Lean nutrient-dense proteins, including fish, poultry, nuts, seeds, and whole grains, should be strongly encouraged.[36]

Protein requires insulin and can increase plasma glucose concentrations. When consuming a mixed meal that contains both carbohydrate and protein, insulin dosing may need to be adjusted, as studies have shown that protein can affect postprandial glycemia.[17,37–39]

Fat type is more significant than total amount of fat for metabolic goals and CVD risk, whereas fat amount is more important in achieving weight and glycemic goals. Several randomized controlled trials, which included patients with type 2 diabetes, have reported that a Mediterranean-style eating pattern, rich in polyunsaturated and monounsaturated fats, can improve blood lipids.[40–42] People with diabetes should be advised to follow the dietary guidelines for the general population for the recommended intakes of saturated fat, dietary cholesterol, and *trans* fat.[36] In addition, when saturated fats are decreased in the diet, they should be replaced with unsaturated fats and not with refined carbohydrates.

In a recent randomized within-subject trial the type of fat had no demonstrated impact on the glycemic response; but the amount of fat did have a significant dose-dependent effect on postprandial glycemia.[43] Dietary fat modulates the postprandial glucose response and delays postprandial hyperglycemia, which may occur 3 hours or more after eating a high fat meal.[38,43,44] Results from these studies also indicate great individual differences in postprandial glycemic response. Because a useful algorithm has not been identified, a careful approach to increasing insulin doses for high-fat and/or high-protein meals is warranted to prevent hypoglycemia. For patients using an insulin pump, delivering part of the bolus immediately and the remainder over a programmed duration of time may provide better insulin coverage for mixed meals.[17]

MICRONUTRIENTS

In the absence of underlying deficiencies, for people with diabetes or without diabetes, there is no robust evidence supporting a glycemic benefit of vitamin/mineral supplements, antioxidants, or herbs.[19] Vitamin D[17] and magnesium[45] supplementation may be of benefit on delaying progression to type 2 diabetes in individuals at high risk, but additional research is needed to define clinical indicators where supplementation may be of benefit and when it may be contraindicated. An analysis of one million participant-data associations of supplements and cardiovascular outcomes found vitamin D and calcium combined increased risk of stroke by 17%, whereas folic acid lowered risk by 20%.[46] No other vitamin, mineral, or antioxidant influenced risk in this trial.[46]

Metformin is associated with vitamin B12 deficiency, so periodic testing of vitamin B12 levels should be considered in patients taking this oral agent, particularly in those with anemia or peripheral neuropathy.[17] Populations at risk for nutritional deficiencies, including older adults, pregnant or lactating women, vegans/vegetarians, and people following low-calorie or low-carbohydrate diets, may require multivitamin/mineral supplementation.[19]

ALCOHOL

Moderate alcohol consumption does not seem to have major negative effects on long-term blood glucose management.[17] Associated acute risks with alcohol intake include hypoglycemia, delayed hypoglycemia (particularly for those using insulin or insulin secretagogues), weight gain, and hyperglycemia with excessive ingestion.[17] These risks need to be communicated to patients who choose to drink, and they should be encouraged to monitor blood glucose frequently when consuming alcohol to minimize such risks.

WEIGHT MANAGEMENT

There is convincing evidence that modest, sustained weight loss can delay the progression from prediabetes to type 2 diabetes and is extremely beneficial for the management of overt diabetes.[20,47,48] Generally, at least a 5% weight loss is needed to achieve favorable outcomes in glycemic control, lipids, and blood pressure for those with type 2 diabetes.[47] Because the clinical benefits of weight loss are progressive, more intensive weight loss goals will maximize benefit and should be encouraged based on patient's ability, feasibility, safety, and support system.[49] Because more than 73% of the nation is overweight or obese,[50] it is not surprising that for many people with type 1 diabetes, excess weight presents clinical challenges as well as for those with type 2.[51]

No single eating pattern has been proved to be consistently superior in achieving and sustaining weight loss in diabetes. An energy deficit, regardless of macronutrient composition, will result in weight loss. Intensive lifestyle intervention programs with frequent follow-up are necessary to change eating behaviors and achieve significant reductions in excess body weight and improve clinical indicators.[51]

DIABETES SELF-MANAGEMENT EDUCATION AND SUPPORT

It is simply unrealistic to expect people with diabetes to make all the necessary diet and lifestyle changes without access to continued services and support. In addition to MNT, diabetes self-management education and support (DSMES) programs provide an evidence-based skill set to empower people with diabetes to confidently make self-management decisions and food choices.[52] The overall objectives of DSMES programs are to support informed decision-making, self-care behaviors, problem solving, and active collaboration with the health care team and to improve clinical outcomes, health status, and quality of life.[52] The American Academy of PAs, the American Association of Nurse Practitioners, the American Association of Diabetes Educators, and others, all recommend that providers refer people with diabetes for DSMES.[53]

The ADA Standards of Care 2022[19] recommends the following critical times for referral to and delivery of DSMES:

1. At diagnosis
2. Annually and/or when not meeting treatment targets
3. When complicating factors (health conditions, physical limitations, emotional factors, or basic living needs) develop that influence self-management
4. When transitions in life and care occur

Data indicate people with diabetes who completed greater than 10 hours of DSMES over the course of 6 to 12 months and, those who participated on an ongoing basis had significant reductions in mortality and A1c.[54,55] Despite evidence that DSMES programs and MNT are cost-effective, have a positive impact on all diabetes-related outcomes, and are typically reimbursed by Medicare and private insures, these services are underused. In the United States, less than 5% of Medicare beneficiaries with diabetes and only 6.8% of those privately insured with diagnosed diabetes have used DSMES services.[56,57] One of the Healthy People 2030 goals is to increase the proportion of people with diabetes who get formal diabetes education; although a slight increase was seen between 2017 and 2019,[58] it is likely that there was a decrease in 2020 as a result of the pandemic. To meet the Healthy People 2030 goal, it is necessary to address both provider and patient barriers to DSMES, which include the following:

- Lack of knowledge about the benefits of DSMES services
- Lack of availability of local DSMES services
- Lack of a perceived need to refer to DSMES
- Confusion about referrals
- Inconvenient DSMES service times or locations (eg, lack of evening or weekend classes)
- Unwillingness to participate in group classes[59]

Primary care providers are vital in linking their patients to MNT and DSMS services to help them sustain behaviors needed to self-manage their diabetes. Therefore, it is necessary to have a clear and efficient referral process. The Centers for Disease Control and Prevention offers a toolkit (https://www.cdc.gov/diabetes/dsmes-toolkit/referrals-participation/overcoming-barriers.html) to promote health care provider referrals and provide resources to assist with the development, promotion, implementation, and sustainability of DSMES services.

SUMMARY

Although research has not identified one ideal diet for all those with diabetes, it does provide overwhelming evidence that food choices and eating patterns will affect glycemia, health goals, and quality of life. Therefore, meal planning must be individualized for each patient considering their health status, resources, personal preferences, motivation, and glycemic targets. The ADA emphasizes that MNT is fundamental in the overall diabetes management plan, and the need for MNT should be reassessed frequently by health care providers in collaboration with their patients across the life-span, with special attention during times of changing health status and life stages. Although the RDN is the primary provider of nutrition counseling and education, it is essential that all members of the health care team are equipped to counter the barrage of deceptive and often dangerous nutrition information that their patients receive from social media.

CLINICS CARE POINTS

- Emphasize nonstarchy vegetables.
- Discourage added sugars and refined grains.
- Recommend whole foods over highly processed foods to the extent possible.
- Reduce overall carbohydrate to improve glycemia.
- An energy deficit, regardless of macronutrient composition, will result in weight loss.
- Individuals with type 1 and type 2 diabetes taking insulin at mealtime should be offered intensive and ongoing education on the need to couple insulin administration with food intake and anticipated physical activity.
- Refer all patients for MNT and DSMES on diagnosis of diabetes.

DISCLOSURE

The author has nothing to disclose.

REFERENCES

1. Fryar CD, Carroll MD, Afful J. Prevalence of overweight, obesity, and severe obesity among adults ages 20 and over: United States, 1960-1962 through 2017-2018. 2020. Available at: https://www.cdc.gov/nchs/data/hestat/obesity-adult-17-18/overweight-obesity-adults-H.pdf. Accessed January 30, 2022.
2. Divers J, Mayer-Davis EJ, Lawrence JM, et al. Trends in incidence of type 1 and type 2 diabetes among youths - selected counties and indian reservations, United States, 2002-2015. MMWR Morb Mortal Wkly Rep 2020;69(6):161–5.
3. Nathan DM, Davidson MB, DeFronzo RA, et al. Impaired fasting glucose and impaired glucose tolerance: implications for care. Diabetes Care 2007;30(3):753–9.
4. Boyle JP, Thompson TJ, Gregg EW, et al. Projection of the year 2050 burden of diabetes in the US adult population: dynamic modeling of incidence, mortality, and prediabetes prevalence. Popul Health Metr 2010;8:29.
5. Rodriguez JE, Campbell KM. Racial and ethnic disparities in prevalence and care of patients with type 2 diabetes. Clin Diabetes 2017;35(1):66–70.
6. Beasley JM, Ho JC, Conderino S, et al. Diabetes and hypertension among South Asians in New York and Atlanta leveraging hospital electronic health records. Diabetol Metab Syndr 2021;13(1):146.
7. Kanaya AM, Wassel CL, Mathur D, et al. Prevalence and correlates of diabetes in South asian indians in the United States: findings from the metabolic syndrome and atherosclerosis in South asians living in america study and the multi-ethnic study of atherosclerosis. Metab Syndr Relat Disord 2010;8(2):157–64.
8. Chiu M, Austin PC, Manuel DG, et al. Deriving ethnic-specific BMI cutoff points for assessing diabetes risk. Diabetes Care 2011;34(8):1741–8.

9. American Diabetes Association. Economic costs of diabetes in the U.S. in 2017. Diabetes Care 2018;41(5):917–28.

10. Nathan DM, Group DER. The diabetes control and complications trial/epidemiology of diabetes interventions and complications study at 30 years: overview. Diabetes Care 2014;37(1):9–16.

11. Turner RC. The U.K. prospective diabetes study: a review. Diabetes Care 1998; 21(Supplement_3):C35–8.

12. Battelino T, Danne T, Bergenstal RM, et al. Clinical targets for continuous glucose monitoring data interpretation: recommendations from the international consensus on time in range. Diabetes Care 2019;42(8):1593–603.

13. Committee ADA. 6. Glycemic targets: standards of medical care in diabetes—2022. Diabetes Care 2021;45(Supplement_1):S83–96.

14. Garber AJ, Abrahamzon MJ, Barzilay JI. Consensus statement by the American Association of Clinical Endocrinologists and American Association of Clinical Endocrinologists and American College of Endocrinology on the Comprehensive type 2 Diabetes Management Algorithm-2017 Executive Summary. Endocr Pract 2017;23(1):207–38.

15. CDC. Diabetes. Stay Healthy Website. Centers for Disease Control and Prevention. Available at: www.cdc.gov/diabetes/managing/health.html. Accessed December 13, 2019.

16. National High Blood Pressure Education Program. The seventh report of the joint national committee on prevention, detection evaluation, and treatment of high blood pressure. National Heart, Lung and Blood Institute. Available at: https://www.ncbi.nlm.nih.gov/books/NBK9630/pdf/Bookshelf_NBK9630.pdf. Accessed January 30, 2022.

17. Evert AB, Dennison M, Gardner CD, et al. Nutrition therapy for adults with diabetes or prediabetes: a consensus report. Diabetes Care 2019;42(5):731–54.

18. Davidson P, Ross T, Castor C. Academy of Nutrition and Dietetics: Revised 2017 standards of practice and standards of professional performance for registered dietitian nutritionists (competent, proficient, and expert) in diabetes care. J Acad Nutr Diet 2018;118(5):932–946 e48.

19. Committee ADA. 5. Facilitating behavior change and well-being to improve health outcomes: standards of medical care in diabetes—2022. Diabetes Care 2021; 45(Supplement_1):S60–82.

20. Franz MJ, MacLeod J, Evert A, et al. Academy of Nutrition and Dietetics Nutrition Practice guideline for type 1 and type 2 diabetes in adults: systematic review of evidence for medical nutrition therapy effectiveness and recommendations for integration into the nutrition care process. J Acad Nutr Diet 2017;117(10): 1659–79.

21. Sun Y, You W, Almeida F, et al. The effectiveness and cost of lifestyle interventions including nutrition education for diabetes prevention: a systematic review and meta-analysis. J Acad Nutr Diet 2017;117(3):404–21.e6.

22. Briggs Early K, Stanley K. Position of the Academy of Nutrition and Dietetics: The role of medical nutrition therapy and registered dietitian nutritionists in the prevention and treatment of prediabetes and type 2 diabetes. J Acad Nutr Diet 2018; 118(2):343–53.

23. Karami A, Dahl A, Turner-McGrievy G, et al. Characterizing diabetes, diet, exercise, and obesity comments on Twitter. Int J Inf Management 2018;38:1–6.

24. Lynn T, Rosati P, Leoni Santos G, et al. Sorting the healthy diet signal from the social media expert noise: preliminary evidence from the healthy diet discourse on

Twitter. Int J Environ Res Public Health 2020;17(22). https://doi.org/10.3390/ijerph17228557.

25. Vosoughi S, Roy D, Aral S. The spread of true and false news online. Science 2018;359(6380):1146–51.

26. Office of the Surgeon General. Publications and Reports of the Surgeon General. Confronting health misinformation: the US surgeon General's advisory on Building a healthy information Environment. US Department of Health and Human Services; 2021. Available at: https://www.hhs.gov/sites/default/files/surgeon-general-misinformation-advisory.pdf. Accessed 29 Feb 2022.

27. Wheeler ML, Dunbar SA, Jaacks LM, et al. Macronutrients, food groups, and eating patterns in the management of diabetes: a systematic review of the literature, 2010. Diabetes Care 2012;35(2):434–45.

28. Institutes of Medicine. Dietary reference intakes for energy, carbohydrate, fiber, fat, fatty acids, cholesterol, protein and amino acids. National Academies Press. Available at: https://www.nap.edu/catalog/10490/dietary-reference-intakes-for-energy-carbohydrate-fiber-fatty-acids-cholesterol-protein-and-amino-acids. Accessed February 3, 2022.

29. Sainsbury E, Kizirian NV, Partridge SR, et al. Effect of dietary carbohydrate restriction on glycemic control in adults with diabetes: A systematic review and meta-analysis. Diabetes Res Clin Pract 2018;139:239–52.

30. van Zuuren EJ, Fedorowicz Z, Kuijpers T, et al. Effects of low-carbohydrate-compared with low-fat-diet interventions on metabolic control in people with type 2 diabetes: a systematic review including GRADE assessments. Am J Clin Nutr 2018;108(2):300–31.

31. Vaz EC, Porfírio GJM, Nunes HRC, et al. Effectiveness and safety of carbohydrate counting in the management of adult patients with type 1 diabetes mellitus: a systematic review and meta-analysis. Arch Endocrinol Metab 2018;62(3):337–45.

32. Liu D, Juanchich M, Sirota M, et al. People overestimate verbal quantities of nutrients on nutrition labels. Food Qual Preference 2019;78:103739.

33. Brand-Miller JC, Stockmann K, Atkinson F, et al. Glycemic index, postprandial glycemia, and the shape of the curve in healthy subjects: analysis of a database of more than 1,000 foods. Am J Clin Nutr 2009;89(1):97–105.

34. Committee ADA. 3. Prevention or delay of type 2 diabetes and associated comorbidities: standards of medical care in diabetes—2022. Diabetes Care 2021; 45(Supplement_1):S39–45.

35. Ley SH, Hamdy O, Mohan V, et al. Prevention and management of type 2 diabetes: dietary components and nutritional strategies. Lancet 2014;383(9933): 1999–2007.

36. U.S. Department of Agriculture and U.S. Department of Health and Human Services. Dietary guidelines for Americans 2020-2025. Available at: https://www.dietaryguidelines.gov/sites/default/files/2020-. Accessed January 30, 2022.

37. Bell KJ, Toschi E, Steil GM, et al. Optimized mealtime insulin dosing for fat and protein in type 1 diabetes: application of a model-based approach to derive insulin doses for open-loop diabetes management. Diabetes Care 2016;39(9):1631–4.

38. Smith TA, Smart CE, Howley PP, et al. For a high fat, high protein breakfast, preprandial administration of 125% of the insulin dose improves postprandial glycaemic excursions in people with type 1 diabetes using multiple daily injections: A cross-over trial. Diabet Med 2021;38(7):e14512.

39. Krebs JD, Arahill J, Cresswell P, et al. The effect of additional mealtime insulin bolus using an insulin-to-protein ratio compared to usual carbohydrate counting

on postprandial glucose in those with type 1 diabetes who usually follow a carbohydrate-restricted diet: a randomized cross-over trial. Diabetes Obes Metab 2018;20(10):2486–9.

40. Bloomfield HE, Koeller E, Greer N, et al. Effects on health outcomes of a Mediterranean diet with no restriction on fat intake: a systematic review and meta-analysis. Ann Intern Med 2016;165(7):491–500.

41. Sacks FM, Lichtenstein AH, Wu JHY, et al. Dietary fats and cardiovascular disease: a presidential advisory from the American Heart Association. Circulation 2017;136(3):e1–23.

42. Estruch R, Ros E, Salas-Salvado J, et al. Primary prevention of cardiovascular disease with a Mediterranean diet. N Engl J Med 2013;368(14):1279–90.

43. Bell KJ, Fio CZ, Twigg S, et al. Amount and Type of dietary fat, postprandial glycemia, and insulin requirements in type 1 diabetes: a randomized within-subject trial. Diabetes Care 2020;43(1):59–66.

44. Bell KJ, Smart CE, Steil GM, et al. Impact of fat, protein, and glycemic index on postprandial glucose control in type 1 diabetes: implications for intensive diabetes management in the continuous glucose monitoring era. Diabetes Care 2015;38(6):1008–15.

45. Veronese N, Watutantrige-Fernando S, Luchini C, et al. Effect of magnesium supplementation on glucose metabolism in people with or at risk of diabetes: a systematic review and meta-analysis of double-blind randomized controlled trials. Eur J Clin Nutr 2016;70(12):1354–9.

46. Khan SU, Khan MU, Riaz H, et al. Effects of nutritional supplements and dietary interventions on cardiovascular outcomes: an umbrella review and evidence map. Ann Intern Med 2019;171(3):190–8.

47. Franz MJ, Boucher JL, Rutten-Ramos S, et al. Lifestyle weight-loss intervention outcomes in overweight and obese adults with type 2 diabetes: a systematic review and meta-analysis of randomized clinical trials. J Acad Nutr Diet 2015; 115(9):1447–63.

48. Raynor HA, Davidson PG, Burns H, et al. Medical nutrition therapy and weight loss questions for the evidence analysis library prevention of type 2 diabetes project: systematic reviews. J Acad Nutr Diet 2017;117(10):1578–611.

49. Lean ME, Leslie WS, Barnes AC, et al. Primary care-led weight management for remission of type 2 diabetes (DiRECT): an open-label, cluster-randomised trial. Lancet 2018;391(10120):541–51.

50. Fryar CD, Carroll MD, Afful J. Prevalence of overweight, obesity, and severe obesity among adults aged 20 and over: United States, 1960–1962 through 2017–2018. NCHS Health E-Stats. 2020.

51. Committee ADA. 8. Obesity and weight management for the prevention and treatment of type 2 diabetes: standards of medical care in diabetes—2022. Diabetes Care 2021;45(Supplement_1):S113–24.

52. Funnell MM, Brown TL, Childs BP, et al. National standards for diabetes self-management education. Diabetes Care 2010;33(Suppl 1):S89–96.

53. Powers MA, Bardsley JK, Cypress M, et al. Diabetes self-management education and support in adults with type 2 diabetes: A consensus report of the American Diabetes Association, the Association of Diabetes Care and Education Specialists, the Academy of Nutrition and Dietetics, the American Academy of Family Physicians, the American Academy of PAs, the American Association of Nurse Practitioners, and the American Pharmacists Association. JAAPA 2020;33(7):1–20.

54. He X, Li J, Wang B, et al. Diabetes self-management education reduces risk of all-cause mortality in type 2 diabetes patients: a systematic review and meta-analysis. Endocrine 2017;55(3):712–31.

55. Chrvala CA, Sherr D, Lipman RD. Diabetes self-management education for adults with type 2 diabetes mellitus: A systematic review of the effect on glycemic control. Patient Educ Couns 2016;99(6):926–43.

56. Strawbridge LM, Lloyd JT, Meadow A, et al. Use of Medicare's diabetes self-management training benefit. Health Educ Behav 2015;42(4):530–8.

57. Strawbridge LM, Lloyd JT, Meadow A, et al. One-year outcomes of diabetes self-management training among medicare beneficiaries newly diagnosed with diabetes. Med Care 2017;55(4):391–7.

58. USDA. Diabetes. Healthy People 2030. U.S. Department of Health and Human Services. Available at: https://health.gov/healthypeople/objectives-and-data/browse-objectives/diabetes. Accessed February 3, 2022.

59. CDC. Overcoming Barriers to Referral and Treatment. Centers for Disease Control and Prevention. Available at: https://www.cdc.gov/diabetes/dsmes-toolkit/referrals-participation/overcoming-barriers.html. Accessed February 3, 2022.

Carbohydrate Counting Primer for Primary Care Providers

Lorraine Laccetti Mongiello, DrPH, RDN, CDE

KEYWORDS

- Basic carbohydrate counting • Advanced carbohydrate counting
- Insulin sensitivity factor • Insulin-to-carbohydrate ratio • Correction dose
- Total daily dose

KEY POINTS

- There are two levels of carbohydrate counting: basic and advanced.
- People with diabetes should receive individualized education on self-monitoring carbohydrate intake to optimize meal timing, food choices, and medication/insulin dose.
- Food literacy, numeracy, and patient interest must be assessed before instruction.
- Carbohydrate counting allows freedom of food choices and greater meal time flexibility while maintaining glycemic control.

INTRODUCTION

In 1922, a 14-year-old boy dying from type 1 diabetes became the first person to receive an injection of insulin,[1] and diabetes was transformed from a death sentence to a chronic condition. Before that, those with diabetes were advised to decrease their sugar and starch intake and a common treatment was to put patients on very strict diets with minimal carbohydrates and very few calories, as low as 450 a day.[2] Case histories from the period show that some physicians prescribed a 70% fat, 8% carbohydrate diet as this could eliminate glycosuria and acidosis, decreased coma, and delay death among children with diabetes.[3] Of course, these diets were not sustainable and it was common for patients to die of starvation.[2]

One hundred years later, people with diabetes are still counting carbohydrates, but restricting them is no longer required for all. Today, carbohydrate counting or "carb counting" is an effective meal-planning technique that can be beneficial to those taking insulin, as well as to those who are not.[4,5] Two levels of carbohydrate counting have been defined: basic and advanced.[6] Patients who master either method of

Clinical Nutrition & Interdisciplinary Health Sciences, New York Institute of Technology, Old Westbury, NY 11568-8000, USA
E-mail address: lmongiel@NYIT.edu

Physician Assist Clin 7 (2022) 655–663
https://doi.org/10.1016/j.cpha.2022.06.007
2405-7991/22/© 2022 Elsevier Inc. All rights reserved.

physicianassistant.theclinics.com

meal planning are able to make appropriate choices from a vast variety of foods that they enjoy.

PATIENT EMPOWERMENT

To facilitate behavior change to improve health outcomes, the American Diabetes Association[7] stresses the importance of collaboration between patients and providers and the use of empowering language that is

- Neutral, nonjudgmental, and based on facts, actions, or physiology/biology;
- Free from stigma;
- Strength-based, respectful, and inclusive and that imparts hope; and
- Person centered ("person with diabetes" is preferred over "diabetic").

In addition to empowering language, patients must be educated to gain the confidence to make autonomous decisions about self-care and diet. The old adage, "give a person a fish and you will feed them for a day, teach a person to fish and you will feed them for a lifetime," applies here. Rather than simply telling the person with diabetes what to eat, or what not to eat, they need to be taught how to discover for themselves what is best for them to choose. A health care team that supports autonomy increases the patient's perceived competence and is predictive of lower A1c levels.[8] Mastering carbohydrate counting is one way to foster patient autonomy and improve glycemic control.[9]

BASIC CARBOHYDRATE COUNTING

Basic carbohydrate counting is a structured meal-planning approach that focuses on consistency in both the timing of meals and the amount of carbohydrates in those meals. It is most useful for people who are not taking insulin or those taking a fixed dose of insulin daily. This method is not reserved only for those with type 1 diabetes, both the American and European clinical guidelines recommend that people with type 2 diabetes receive individualized education on self-monitoring carbohydrate intake to optimize meal timing and food choices based on their current dietary intake and glucose-lowering medications.[10,11]

Carbohydrate counting education involves teaching patients the relationship among food intake, oral antihyperglycemic medications, insulin, physical activity, and blood glucose (BG) levels. With this approach, a set amount of carbohydrates is consumed at each meal and, if necessary, with snacks. It is important to note that, whereas the grams of carbohydrate consumed should remain fairly constant from day to day[5] the variety of food should not.

A shortcoming of this method is that variations in physical activity are more likely to cause high- or low BG levels because the patient is not adjusting food intake or insulin dose to compensate for changes in activity. Guidance is required to reduce this risk for those using insulin or insulin secretagogues.

The initial challenge is to determine a patient's "carb allowance" for each meal. As one's tolerance for carbohydrates is extremely variable, there is no formula to accurately ascertain optimal intake. It is best determined by assessment of current intake and glycemia. This entails keeping detailed food intake records and pre-/post-meal BG logs. The patient must be able to identify all sources of carbohydrates, read food labels, and weigh and measure foods accurately. This can be facilitated by one of the many available food tracking applications. Together, the patient with diabetes and the educator must review the data collected to determine carbohydrate limits based on postprandial glycemia. The American College of Clinical

Endocrinology recommends a 2-h postprandial glycemic target of 140 mg/dL for nonpregnant adults.[12] An after-meal BG rise of about 40 mg/dL would generally indicate that an adequate amount of food was consumed.

Table 1 provides a sample food and BG record. At first glance, it may appear to the patient that BG levels vary from day to day in an unpredictable way. It would also likely be assumed that the breakfast on day 3 was a poor choice because it resulted in the highest postprandial glucose level. Teaching the patient to identify and calculate the amount of carbohydrates in a meal allows for a more accurate and useful interpretation of the data they collect.

In **Table 2**, the amount of carbohydrate consumed and the change in BG have been calculated by the dietitian. It now becomes evident that the sandwich eaten on day 3 provided 44 g of carbohydrate and only increased BG by 27 points. It is likely that the elevated level of 185 mg/dL was due to a high pre-meal level, not the food choice. On day 4, a very high carbohydrate meal was consumed, which accounts for the biggest increase in glycemia. While on day 2, only 15 g of carbohydrate was ingested resulting in only a slight increase. The patient would need to be made aware that, whereas this meal did not negatively impact his or her BG level, it is high in saturated fat and low in fiber. Based on these records, it can be estimated that the patient's "carb allowance" for breakfast would be approximately 55 g as this amount kept him or her in the target range, whereas 44 g was too little and, clearly 108 g was too much. This allowance would then need to be tested and, if necessary, adjusted. By limiting intake to this amount of carbohydrate, regardless of type, target goals will likely be achieved.

ADVANCED CARBOHYDRATE COUNTING

Instead of being based on a structured approach and consistency, advanced carbohydrate counting involves matching a variable dose of insulin to the amount of carbohydrate desired at each meal. Thus, carbohydrates can vary in both type and amount from meal to meal and from day to day. The ADA Standards of Medical Care in Diabetes–2022 states that individuals with type 1 or type 2 diabetes, taking insulin at meal time, should be offered intensive advanced carbohydrate counting training and ongoing education to teach them how to match insulin dosing with carbohydrate intake.[13]

Whereas this method ultimately simplifies food decisions for those with diabetes, initially it can be daunting. Food literacy, numeracy, patient interest, and capability must be assessed to determine if they are a good candidate for advanced carbohydrate counting. Specific strategies might be required for patients with a lower level of education and with a history or current depression considering their likely lower perceived level of confidence.[14] The incorporation of technology, such as continuous glucose monitoring (CGM), insulin pumps with bolus algorithms, and telemedicine can be efficacious in improving confidence, accuracy, and outcomes.[15]

Table 1
Food and blood glucose log for patient not requiring insulin

Patient Log 1	Day 1	Day 2	Day 3	Day 4
Premeal BG	105 mg/dL	98 mg/dL	154 mg/dL	95 mg/dL
Meal	1 cup corn flakes 8 oz. 1% milk 1 cup blueberries	2 hardboiled eggs 3 slices bacon 1 slice bread 1 tbsp. butter	Panera veggie on tomato basil sandwich	1 seeded bagel 8 oz. orange juice 6 oz. fruit yogurt
2 h Postmeal BG	139 mg/dL	119 mg/dL	185 mg/dL	165mg/dL

Table 2
Food, blood glucose and carbohydrate log for patient not requiring insulin

Patient Log 2	Day 1	Day 2	Day 3	Day 4
Pre-meal BG	101 mg/dL	98 mg/dL	158 mg/dL	94 mg/dL
Meal	1 cup corn flakes 8 oz. 1% milk 1 cup blueberries	2 hardboiled eggs 3 slices bacon 1 slice bread 1 tbsp. butter	Panera veggie on tomato basil sandwich	1 seeded bagel 8 oz. orange juice 6 oz. fruit yogurt
Carbohydrate	54 g	15 g	44 g	108 g
2-h Post-meal BG	139 mg/dL	109 mg/dL	185 mg/dL	165mg/dL
BG change	↑ 38 mg/dL	↑ 11 mg/dL	↑ 27 mg/dL	↑ 71 mg/dL

Step 1: Cover the Carbohydrates

To cover the total grams of carbohydrate in a meal the patient's insulin-to-carbohydrate ratio (ICR) must be determined. This ratio may be 1:15 for someone who is very sensitive to insulin or only 1:5 for someone who is less sensitive. A ratio of 1:10, for example, indicates that for every 10 g of carbohydrate consumed, 1 unit of rapid-acting insulin is required. Note that if a portion of food has $\geq$5 g of either fiber or sugar alcohol per serving half the amount of each should be subtracted from the total grams of carbohydrate in the item.

Example: A slice of bread containing 22 g of total carbohydrate and 6 g of fiber would be counted as proving 19 g of carbohydrate.

$6/2 = 3$; $22-3 = 19$.

A starting ICR can be estimated based on a person's weight (ie, 101–120 lbs. −1:18; 231–270 lbs. −1:6). This approach is based on the general observation that insulin resistance increases as body size increases. Thus, each unit of insulin will cover more carbohydrates in a lighter person than in a heavier person. A potential problem with this method is that it does not consider body composition. An individual who weighs 200 pounds, but is very muscular, will be much more sensitive to insulin than a 200-pound person with a great deal of body fat. It is also important to note that generally, one's sensitivity to insulin increases during the day. This makes it possible that ICR will vary from breakfast to dinner and basing the ratio on weight alone will not account for this.

A second way to approximate a starting ICR is the "500 rule," which is based on the premise that people consume about 500 g of carbohydrates daily. To determine ICR using this method simply divide 500 by a patient's total daily dose (TDD) of both basal and bolus insulin.

Example: If the patient is currently injecting 15 units of long-acting insulin and 25 units of rapid-acting insulin daily, the starting ICR is 1:12.5.

TDD: $15 + 25 = 40$ units

$500/40 = 12.5$

Three major weaknesses of the 500 rule are (1) it assumes that all people eat about the same amount of carbohydrates daily, (2) it assumes the current TDD of insulin is adequately controlling BG, and (3) it does not take into account the changes in insulin sensitivity throughout the day. Both the 500 rule and the weight method require trial and error and fine-tuning to ascertain precise ICRs.

Alternately, ICRs can better be determined by reviewing food logs, which include accurate recording of intake, insulin dose, and pre/postmeal BG levels. CGM is extremely useful in this process, but the task can be accomplished with self-monitoring of BG as well. While this process can be tedious and requires frequent sessions with the educator, a learning-by-doing model (problem-based and experience-based patient education) supports the development of the necessary skills and can improve diet quality overall.[16,17]

Table 3 provides very useful data from a patient currently on a fixed dose of insulin regardless of food intake. The consistency of insulin coupled with the inconsistency of meals resulted in a great variation of day-to-day postprandial glucose levels. In this case, on days 1 and 4 insulin dose was most accurate as evidenced by a postprandial excursion of about 40 mg/dL or less. Whereas on day 2, too much insulin was injected, and on day 3 too little. By calculating the ICR that was used on each of these days it can be determined that an ICR of 1:12 would be a good starting point. This ratio would then need to be tested and fine-tuned by continuing to analyze the patient's logs at varying times of a day to evaluate individual responses and guide insulin dose adjustments. Once established, the ICR can be applied to both high and low carbohydrate meals and less glucose testing would be required.

Protein and Fat

For more precise insulin dosing the amount of protein and fat may also need to be considered.[13,18,19] However, studies point to individual differences in the postprandial glycemic response of mixed meals and more research needs to be done to determine a useful algorithm.[20–23] Thus, the effects of protein and high-fat meals should be addressed as they arise and should be considered a need-to-know tool that can be taught to patients who may benefit from using it based on their eating patterns and BG data.[18]

We do know:

- Protein influences postprandial glycemia and this effect is likely delayed by approximately 1.5 hours.[24]
- High-fat meals, such as pizza or fast food, can cause delayed and/or prolonged hyperglycemia up to 35 hours after eating.[20]
- A cautious approach to increasing insulin doses for high-fat and/or high-protein mixed meals is recommended to prevent both hypoglycemia and delayed hyperglycemia.[18]
- If using an insulin pump, a split bolus feature (part of the bolus delivered immediately, the remainder over a programmed duration of time) may provide better insulin coverage for high-fat and/or high-protein mixed meals.[18]

Step 2: Apply Correction Dose

Using the correct ICR will cover a meal, but it will not correct for high or low pre-meal BG. Therefore, the premeal insulin dose must be adjusted if BG is out of range. This is

Table 3
Insulin dose, carbohydrate intake, and blood glucose log for patient with TY1 DM

Patient Log 3	Day 1	Day 2	Day 3	Day 4
Pre-Meal BG	105 mg/dL	98 mg/dL	100 mg/dL	95 mg/dL
Rapid insulin dose	5 units	5 units	5 units	5 units
Carbohydrate intake	62 g	28 g	82 g	55 g
2-h Post-meal BG	142 mg/dL	76 mg/dL	189 mg/dL	120/mg dL
BG change	↑ 37 mg/dL	↓22 mg/dL	↑ 89 mg/dL	↑ 25 mg/dL
Target achieved	Yes	No	No	Yes
ICR (carbohydrate/insulin)	62/5 = 12.4	28/5 = 5.6	82/5 = 16.4	55/5 = 11

Nutrition Facts

8 servings per container

Serving size   2/3 cup (55g)

Amount per serving

Calories   230

	% Daily Value*
Total Fat 8g	**10%**
Saturated Fat 1g	**5%**
Trans Fat 0g	
Cholesterol 0mg	**0%**
Sodium 160mg	**7%**
Total Carbohydrate 37g	**13%**
Dietary Fiber 4g	**14%**
Total Sugars 12g	
Includes 10g Added Sugars	**20%**
Protein 3g	
Vitamin D 2mcg	10%
Calcium 260mg	20%
Iron 8mg	45%
Potassium 240mg	6%

Fig. 1. Carbohydrate counting primer for primary care providers. Changes to the Nutrition Facts Label, U.S. Food and Drug Administration. https://www.fda.gov/food/food-labeling-nutrition/changes-nutrition-facts-label. [a]The % Daily Value (DV) tells you how much a nutrient in a serving food of contributes to a daily diet. 2,000 calories a day is used for general nutrition diet.

achieved by determining the insulin sensitivity factor (ISF), sometimes called a correction factor. The ISF is simply a measure of the amount by which BG is reduced by one unit of rapid-acting insulin in a period of 2–4 hours. Generally, one unit of rapid insulin is needed to drop BG by 50 mg/dL. However, this drop in BG can range from 30 mg/dL to 100 mg/dL, depending on individual insulin sensitivities and other circumstances.

The standard "1700 rule" is used to estimate an ISF with rapid-acting insulin. Simply divide 1700 by the TDD of insulin. If the TDD is 55 units, then the ISF is 31 (1700/55). The ISF is fine-tuned, based on results, and applied when premeal BG is either above or below target.

Example:

BG—188 mg/dL

Target BG—95 mg/dL

Carbohydrate—48 g

ISF—31

ICR—12

In this case, the appropriate insulin dose would be 7 units of rapid-acting insulin. To cover the carbohydrate, 4 units are required (48/12 = 4) and an additional 3 units are needed to correct the premeal hyperglycemia as glucose was 93 points above target. (93/31 = 3).

It is important to consider how much insulin is on board before applying a correction dose to prevent insulin stacking. This occurs when a dose of rapid-acting insulin is given while a previous insulin dose is still active, this increases the potential for severe hypoglycemia. Stacking is less likely with insulin pumps because they can take into account active insulin when calculating a bolus dose. Additionally, several useful applications are available that calculate an insulin dose based on carbohydrate intake, a person's IRC, correction factor, and target BG levels.[9,25]

A potential drawback of carbohydrate counting, both basic and advanced, is overconsumption. Since the focus is solely on carbohydrates and portions are not limited, patients may eat too many calories and overlook the amount and type of fat they're consuming. Weight and lipid levels need to be monitored and, when necessary, nutrition education and support are to be provided to reinforce eating patterns that align with the US Dietary Guidelines.[26]

SUMMARY

Carbohydrates, both sugars and starches, greatly affect postprandial BG levels. Protein and fats have a much lesser effect but can delay or prolong hyperglycemia depending on the amount consumed. Both basic and advanced carbohydrate counting are effective meal-planning strategies to achieve glycemic targets. They also empower patients by allowing freedom of food choices and greater meal-time flexibility. A variety of self-management skills is necessary to successfully implement carbohydrate counting, requiring the need for ongoing education and support to ensure success.[13]

CLINICS CARE POINTS

- The American College of Clinical Endocrinology recommends a 2-h postprandial glycemic target of 140 mg/dL for nonpregnant adults.
- Clinical guidelines recommend that people with type 1 and type 2 diabetes receive individualized education on carbohydrate counting to optimize food choices, foster patient autonomy, and improve glycemic control.
- For those taking insulin at meal time, intensive advanced carbohydrate counting training and ongoing education to teach them how to match insulin dosing with carbohydrate intake should be provided.
- For more precise insulin dosing the amount of protein and fat may also need to be considered if targets are not achieved based on carbohydrate intake alone.
- A cautious approach to increasing insulin doses for high-fat and/or high-protein mixed meals is recommended to prevent both hypoglycemia and delayed hyperglycemia.

CLINICAL QUESTION

Your patient's current BG is 180 mg/dL and she is planning to have 1 cup of the food described in **Fig. 1**. Her ICR is 15, ISF is 35, and her premeal BG target is 100 mg/dL. How much rapid-acting insulin should she administer before the meal?

Answer
- Patient requires 6 units of rapid-acting insulin.

Explanation

Step 1—Cover the Carbohydrates
- There are 55.5 g of carbohydrate in one cup of this food.
- There are 6 g of fiber in one cup of this food.
- Subtract half the fiber from total carbohydrate: 55.5 − 3 = 52.5.
- 52.5/15 = 3.7 units are needed to cover the meal.

Step 2—Correct Pre-meal Hyperglycemia
- Patient is 80 points above target.
- 80/35 = 2.3 units are needed for correction.

3.7 + 2.3 = 6 units

DISCLOSURE

The author has nothing to disclose.

REFERENCES

1. Banting FG, Best CH, Collip JB, et al. Pancreatic extracts in the treatment of diabetes mellitus. Can Med Assoc J 1922;12(3):141–6.
2. Mazur A. Why were "starvation diets" promoted for diabetes in the pre-insulin period? Nutr J 2011;10:23.
3. Westman EC, Yancy WS, Humphreys M. Dietary treatment of diabetes mellitus in the pre-insulin era (1914-1922). Perspect Biol Med 2006;49(1):77–83.
4. Vaz EC, Porfírio GJM, Nunes HRC, et al. Effectiveness and safety of carbohydrate counting in the management of adult patients with type 1 diabetes mellitus: a systematic review and meta-analysis. Arch Endocrinol Metab 2018;62(3):337–45.
5. Franz MJ, MacLeod J, Evert A, et al. Academy of Nutrition and Dietetics nutrition practice guideline for type 1 and type 2 diabetes in adults: systematic review of evidence for medical nutrition therapy effectiveness and recommendations for integration into the nutrition care process. J Acad Nutr Diet 2017;117(10):1659–79.
6. Gillespie SJ, Kulkarni KD, Daly AE. Using carbohydrate counting in diabetes clinical practice. J Am Diet Assoc 1998;98(8):897–905.
7. Committee ADA. 4. Comprehensive medical evaluation and assessment of comorbidities: standards of medical care in diabetes—2022. Diabetes Care 2021;45(Supplement_1):S46–59.
8. Williams GC, Freedman ZR, Deci EL. Supporting autonomy to motivate patients with diabetes for glucose control. Diabetes Care 1998;21(10):1644–51.
9. Christensen MB, Serifovski N, Herz AMH, et al. Efficacy of bolus calculation and advanced carbohydrate counting in type 2 diabetes: a randomized clinical trial. Diabetes Technol Ther 2021;23(2):95–103.
10. Davies MJ, D'Alessio DA, Fradkin J, et al. Management of hyperglycaemia in type 2 diabetes, 2018. A consensus report by the American Diabetes Association (ADA) and the European Association for the Study of Diabetes (EASD). Diabetologia 2018;61(12):2461–98. https://doi.org/10.1007/s00125-018-4729-5.
11. Holt RIG, DeVries JH, Hess-Fischl A, et al. The management of type 1 diabetes in adults. A consensus report by the American Diabetes Association (ADA) and the European Association for the Study of Diabetes (EASD). Diabetologia 2021;64(12):2609–52.
12. Garber AJ, Abrahamzon MJ, Barzilay JI. Consensus statement by the American Association of Clinical Endocrinologists and American Association of Clinical Endocrinologists and American College of Endocrinology on the comprehensive type 2 diabetes management algorithm-2017 executive summary. Endocr Pract 2017;23(1):207–38.
13. Committee ADA. 5. Facilitating behavior change and well-being to improve health outcomes: standards of medical care in diabetes—2022. Diabetes Care 2021;45(Supplement_1):S60–82.

14. Fortin A, Rabasa-Lhoret R, Roy-Fleming A, et al. Practices, perceptions and expectations for carbohydrate counting in patients with type 1 diabetes - results from an online survey. Diabetes Res Clin Pract 2017;126:214–21.
15. Committee ADA. 7. Diabetes technology: standards of medical care in diabetes—2022. Diabetes Care 2021;45(Supplement_1):S97–112.
16. McGowan L, Caraher M, Raats M, et al. Domestic cooking and foodskills: a review. Sci Nutr 2017;57:2412–31.
17. Hill-Briggs F, Lazo M, Peyrot M, et al. Effect of problem-solving-based diabetes self-management training on diabetes control in a low income patient sample. J Gen Intern Med 2011;26(9):972–8.
18. Evert AB, Dennison M, Gardner CD, et al. Nutrition therapy for adults with diabetes or prediabetes: a consensus report. Diabetes Care 2019;42(5):731–54.
19. Smart CEM, King BR, Lopez PE. Insulin dosing for fat and protein: is it time? Diabetes Care 2020;43(1):13–5.
20. Bell KJ, Fio CZ, Twigg S, et al. Amount and type of dietary fat, postprandial glycemia, and insulin requirements in type 1 diabetes: a randomized within-subject trial. Diabetes Care 2020;43(1):59–66.
21. Bell KJ, Smart CE, Steil GM, et al. Impact of fat, protein, and glycemic index on postprandial glucose control in type 1 diabetes: implications for intensive diabetes management in the continuous glucose monitoring era. Diabetes Care 2015;38(6):1008–15.
22. Furthner D, Lukas A, Schneider AM, et al. The role of protein and fat intake on insulin therapy in glycaemic control of pediatric type 1 diabetes: a systematic review and research gaps. Nutrients 2021;13(10):3558.
23. Krebs JD, Arahill J, Cresswell P, et al. The effect of additional mealtime insulin bolus using an insulin-to-protein ratio compared to usual carbohydrate counting on postprandial glucose in those with type 1 diabetes who usually follow a carbohydrate-restricted diet: a randomized cross-over trial. Diabetes Obes Metab 2018;20(10):2486–9.
24. Paterson MA, Smart CEM, Lopez PE, et al. Increasing the protein quantity in a meal results in dose-dependent effects on postprandial glucose levels in individuals with Type 1 diabetes mellitus. Diabet Med 2017;34(6):851–4. https://doi.org/10.1111/dme.13347.
25. Hommel E, Schmidt S, Vistisen D, et al. Effects of advanced carbohydrate counting guided by an automated bolus calculator in type 1 diabetes mellitus (StenoABC): a 12-month, randomized clinical trial. Diabet Med 2017;34(5):708–15.
26. U.S. Department of Agriculture and U.S Department of Health and Human Services. Dietary guidelines for Americans 2020-2025. Available at: https://www.dietaryguidelines.gov/sites/default/files/2020-. Accessed February 27, 2022.

Obesity, Bariatric Surgery, and Postoperative Nutritional Management

Jill R. Silverman, PhD, RDN

KEYWORDS

- Bypass • Duodenal switch • Gastric sleeve • Weight loss • BMI • Diet
- Malabsorption

KEY POINTS

- 40% of American adults are diagnosed with obesity.
- 90% of people who lose weight through lifestyle changes alone, regain the weight.
- Bariatric surgeries provide sustainable weight loss and, in many cases, a resolution of type 2 diabetes and other obesity-related diseases.
- Postsurgery, lifelong compliance to dietary and behavioral modification is required.

INTRODUCTION

The diet industry accrued $71 billion in 2020, yet over 42% of American adults have obesity, a chronic disease state associated with type 2 diabetes, coronary vascular disease, and sleep apnea. With a reported 80–95% of people regaining weight lost through diet and exercise alone, it is important to consider alternative strategies for sustainable weight loss. Bariatric surgeries result in maintainable weight loss due to a significant reduction in food intake and inhibition of energy absorption. However, continued success requires a lifetime commitment to behavior modification and dietary compliance.

EPIDEMIOLOGY OF OBESITY

Obesity, a chronic disease categorized as a body mass index (BMI) greater than 30, affects 4 in 10 adults in the US. Chronic disease states associated with excess weight include type 2 diabetes, hypertension, heart disease, sleep apnea, and certain cancers. Obesity is the second most common preventable cause of premature death (after smoking) in the US.[1,2] In addition, obesity is associated with an increased risk of COVID-19–related complications.[3]

Department of Nutrition Science, Farmingdale State College, 2350 Broadhollow Road, Farmingdale, NY 11735, USA
E-mail address: silverj@farmingdale.edu

Physician Assist Clin 7 (2022) 665–683
https://doi.org/10.1016/j.cpha.2022.06.006
physicianassistant.theclinics.com

DEMOGRAPHICS AND COST OF OBESITY

Obesity is most prevalent among 40- to 59-year-old adults (44.8%) and age-adjusted non-Hispanic Black adults (49.6%).[4] In 2016, the estimated annual direct costs (medical care) of obesity in the US were $480.7 billion. Indirect costs (the loss of productivity due to obesity-related absenteeism) were approximately $1.72 trillion.[5,6]

DISCUSSION
Nonsurgical Treatment of Obesity

Diet and exercise
Hippocrates said, "If we could give every individual the right amount of nourishment and exercise, not too little and not too much, we would have found the safest way to health." This pretty much sums up the approach to weight loss in the 20th century. However, it is now known that there is more to the treatment of obesity than calories in < calories out and will power. Other factors include genetics, epigenetics, leptin resistance, adipocytokines, intrauterine effects, gut microbiota, and an obesogenic environment.[7,8] It has been demonstrated that diets and physical activity alone do not lead to long-term weight loss for the majority of people; roughly 85% of people regain the weight lost through diet and exercise after a year.[9] Proposed mechanisms for the reported weight regain are a reduction in metabolic rate that accompanies weight loss, and the body's predisposition to compensate for weight loss by increasing appetite and decreasing energy expenditure, to maintain the body's inherent weight set point.[10–12]

Weight loss drugs
Pharmacotherapy is another weight loss strategy utilized concurrently with diet and exercise. Current FDA-approved weight loss medications for long-term use include the appetite suppressants: Bupropion-naltrexone (Contrave), Liraglutide (Saxenda), Phentermine-topiramate (Qsymia), and Wegovy (Semaglutide), and the lipase inhibitor Orlistat (Xenical), which is also available over the counter as Alli, a reduced strength form.[13,14] Most of these medications result in a modest weight loss of 5–10% of a patient's starting weight.[15,16] Pharmacotherapy combined with diet, exercise, and behavioral modification results in an increased likelihood of maintaining weight loss after 1 year. However, weight regain often occurs when medication is stopped.[17]

Surgical Treatment of Obesity

Criteria for surgery
As mentioned above, bariatric surgeries are associated with significant and maintainable weight loss. Typically, before being considered a candidate for bariatric surgery, a person will have attempted other weight loss strategies, without long-term success. Additional prerequisites for most weight loss surgeries include being at least 18 years of age, having a BMI ≥40, 100 pounds over the recommended weight, or having a BMI ≥35 and an obesity-related medical condition such as sleep apnea, diabetes, high cholesterol, or blood pressure.[18]

Preoperative nutrition management
One to two weeks prior to surgery, to reduce liver size and facilitate the surgery and recuperation, the patient will transition to a low-fat, mostly liquid diet consisting of protein drinks, to ensure adequate intake of their daily protein requirement (60–80 grams). Other permitted liquids include water, caffeine-free coffee and teas, low sodium broths, and sugar-free, noncarbonated beverages, popsicles, and gelatin. Small

servings of fish, low-fat dairy, watered-down hot cereals, and eggs may be allowed. It is especially important, not only presurgery but postsurgery (**Table 1**), as well, to consume the required 64 ounces of fluids daily.[19]

Mechanisms and frequency of procedures

Bariatric procedures lead to weight loss by restricting caloric intake, and/or decreasing the absorption of calories (malabsorption). Restrictive procedures decrease stomach size resulting in a reduction in the volume of food able to be ingested. These include the adjustable gastric band (AGB), laparoscopic sleeve gastrectomy (LSG), and the intragastric balloon (IGB). Malabsorptive procedures result in a decrease in nutrient absorption due to the removal of a portion of the small intestine. Gastric bypass (GB), biliopancreatic diversion with duodenal switch (BDS-DS), and single anastomosis duodenal-ileal bypass with sleeve gastrectomy (SADI-S) use a combination of both retriction and malabsorption for weight loss .[20,21] In 2011, out of the 158,000 weight loss surgeries performed, 17.8%, 36.7%, and 35.4% were LSG, GB, and AGB procedures, respectively. Of the 278,000 weight loss surgeries performed in 2019, the majority were LSG (59.4%) followed by GB (17.8%).[22] Bariatric surgery is performed laparoscopically, due to fewer surgical complications, than open surgery.[23–25]

Types of surgery

- *Adjustable gastric band*

The AGB surgery involves the insertion of an inflatable balloon-containing band around the top of the stomach creating a small pouch, restricting the amount of food a person needs to consume before experiencing fullness (**Fig. 1**).[26]

At subsequent office visits, additional saline can be added to the adjustable band through an injection port located under the skin, reducing the size of the orifice between the pouch and the remainder of the stomach , thereby slowing the rate of gastric emptying. Therefore, the subsequent satiety and weight loss experienced after AGB surgery are not only due to a restriction in stomach capacity but to a delay in gastric emptying, as well. Patients must adhere to a diet of small meals and avoid calorically dense beverages which can pass straight through the orifice, without contributing to satiety. In addition, foods need to be consumed slowly and chewed thoroughly to avoid blocking the opening. In recent years, the AGB has not been a preferred procedure (down from 35.4% in 2011 to 0.9% in 2019)[28] due to its higher rate of postsurgical complications (**Table 2**) and slower weight loss compared to other bariatric surgeries. Subsequently, many patients have the AGB removed.[29]

- Laparoscopic sleeve gastrectomy

LSG is typically performed as the first step in the BPD-DS. However, significant weight loss was observed among patients after undergoing LSG alone, so it is now used as a distinct weight loss surgery for the treatment of obesity. In addition to resulting in significant, maintainable weight loss, LSG is associated with a reduction in obesity-related morbidities.[30–32] As seen in **Fig. 2**, LSG involves the permanent removal of approximately 75% of the stomach with the remaining quarter stapled into the form of a banana-shaped tube or sleeve.

In addition to early satiety, a result of reduced stomach capacity, the procedure prompts a decrease in the level of the gut-produced hormone, ghrelin ("the hunger hormone"), resulting in increased appetite suppression.[33] In addition to weight loss,

Table 1
General requirements and restrictions following bariatric surgery. Recommendations may differ depending on the surgery and surgery center[19,48-51]

Approximate Duration Stage	Recommended Amount to Consume	Permitted Foods	Avoid
2 weeks *Full liquids*	No more than: 2 Tablespoons at a time 400 calories/day	Same as preoperative diet recommendations 64 ounces of fluids between meals High protein, including protein supplements	Fat Sugar Alcohol Caffeine Carbonated beverages Straws
2 weeks *Blended foods* - pureed to baby food consistency	No more than: one-fourth cup solid food/meal 500 calories/day	Protein-rich foods: lean ground meats, fish, eggs, low-fat dairy, cottage cheese, yogurt, tofu, hummus 64 ounces of fluids between meals High protein, including protein supplements Multivitamin and mineral supplements	Same as above AND Empty calorie foods Adding liquids to foods (will dilute nutrients)
4 weeks *Soft, easy-to-chew foods*	Same as blended food stage	Same as above but foods do not need to be pureed AND Nonstarchy vegetables: cooked and raw (as tolerated)	Same as above
Lifelong *General diet*	Small, frequent meals No more than: 800–1000 calories/day	Same as above AND Fruits without skin 6 months postsurgery, patient can add *limited* amounts daily of: complex carbohydrates: brown rice, beans, quinoa, steel-cut oatmeal, lentils, whole wheat bread, sweet potato, bulgur, barley Caffeinated beverages (do not contribute to daily liquid requirements) Alcoholic beverages (do not contribute to daily liquid requirements)	Straws Empty calorie foods Refined carbohydrates Calorically dense beverages High-fat foods Carbonated beverages Adding liquids to foods(will dilute nutrients)

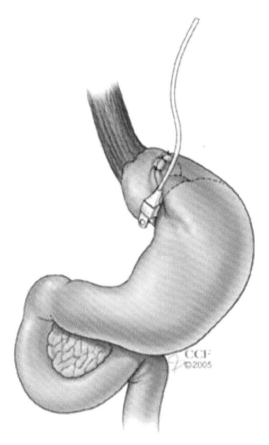

Fig. 1. Adjustable gastric band. (*Adapted from* the American Society for Bariatric and Metabolic Surgery[27]; with permission.)

LSG is associated with an improvement in glycemic control and resolution of diabetes in over 60% of patients.[34]

- Gastric bypass

In GB or the Roux-en-Y (Fr: in the form of a Y) procedure, the stomach capacity is permanently reduced to a 1-ounce gastric pouch, resulting in increased satiety. The newly formed restrictive pouch is then attached to a lower portion of the small intestine, bypassing the absorptive surface of the duodenum and first part of the jejunum (**Fig. 3**).

The result is a reduction in the absorption of nutrients from food, yielding fewer calories in the body and, subsequently, weight loss. The bypassed portion of the stomach and duodenum are attached further down the small intestine resulting in a bowel connection resembling the letter Y.[35] In addition to weight loss, GB results in the improvement or remission of type 2 diabetes in approximately 80% of patients.[36]

- Biliopancreatic diversion with duodenal switch

The BPD-DS is typically used for patients with a BMI ≥50 or a BMI of ≥40 and a serious obesity-related condition. It may also be used as a successive operation for patients who underwent LSG with unsatisfactory weight loss. As seen in **Fig. 4**, the

Table 2
Long-term outcomes, advantages, and disadvantages of different bariatric surgeries

Surgery	Average Percent Excess Weight Lost (when Combined with Lifestyle Changes)	Pros	Cons
AGB	40	Minimally invasive Reversible Adjustable	Band deterioration or slippage Unsatisfactory weight loss High rates of reoperation No improvement of type 2 diabetes
LSG	60	Minimally invasive Reduced amount of food intake while preserving normal gastrointestinal tract functions Fewer food intolerances	Not reversible or adjustable Stretching of the sleeve Stapling complications Stenosis/Strictures Bleeding Increased incidence of gastroesophageal reflux disease (GERD)
GB	70	Reliable, long-lasting weight loss Resolution of obesity-related conditions	Technically more complex when compared to ASB and LSG Increased risk of malabsorption and potential deficiencies than ASB or LSG Risk of ulcers and small bowel obstruction Dumping syndrome[a] Increased incidence of GERD
BPD-DS	70–80	Among the best results for improving obesity Affects bowel hormones to cause less hunger and more fullness after eating Most effective procedure for the treatment of type 2 diabetes	Higher complication rates than other procedures – involves 2 intestinal fusions Highest malabsorption rate - greater possibility of nutrient deficiencies Risk of looser and more frequent bowel movements Increased incidence of (GERD)

SADI-S	80	Highly effective for long-term weight loss and remission of type 2 diabetes Simpler and faster to perform (1 intestinal connection) than gastric bypass or BPD-DS Excellent option for a patient who had sleeve gastrectomy and is seeking further weight loss	Increased malabsorption and potential deficiencies than ASB or LSG Newer operation with only short-term outcome data Risk of looser and more frequent bowel movements Development of GERD
IGB	29	Noninvasive Available to patients who may not be eligible for weight loss surgery.	Weight regain if lifestyle changes are not maintained once IGB is removed

[a] *Dumping syndrome* occurs when foods high in sugar or fat are consumed too quickly or in too large a quantity. The food is "dumped" into the small intestine before being properly digested in the stomach. Dumping syndrome is associated with nausea, cramping, diarrhea, sweating, vomiting, or an increase in heart rate and can last up to two hours. Patients can reduce the risk of dumping syndrome by avoiding foods high in sugar and fat, eating slowly, and chewing foods thoroughly.([29,45,46,77–86]).

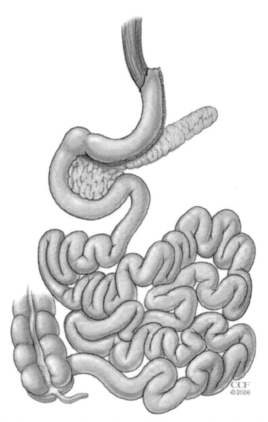

Fig. 2. Laparoscopic sleeve gastrectomy. (*Adapted from* the American Society for Bariatric and Metabolic Surgery[27]; with permission.)

BPD-DS is a two-step process beginning with the permanent removal of 75% of the stomach, creating a restrictive tube-shaped stomach (gastric sleeve). Next, the newly created sleeve is attached to the ileum, so that approximately two-thirds of the intestine is bypassed (the duodenal switch), resulting in a significant decrease in nutrients absorbed and calories yielded by the body.[37,38]

Like LSG and GB, the significant weight loss reported from the BPD-DS is associated not only with changes in the gastrointestinal anatomy but with altered levels of gut hormones, resulting in reduced hunger and increased fullness. In addition, the most substantial improvement in blood sugar levels is observed among patients with BPD-DS; more than 85% remission.[39,40]

- Single anastomosis duodenal-ileal bypass with sleeve gastrectomy

The SADI-S, although similar to the BPD-DS, is a less complicated and shorter surgery as only one intestinal connection is required instead of two. After the capacity of the stomach is permanently restricted through the formation of a gastric sleeve, it is connected to the last several feet of the small intestine. Therefore, upon consumption, food goes through the sleeve and directly into the latter portion of the small intestine, bypassing the majority of the intestine's absorptive surface. The food then mixes with digestive juices from the first part of the small intestine (**Fig. 5**).[41–43]

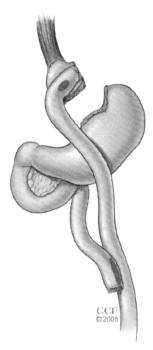

Fig. 3. Roux-en-Y gastric bypass. (*Adapted from* the American Society for Bariatric and Metabolic Surgery[27]; with permission.)

After surgery, in addition to weight loss, patients experience less hunger, increased satiety, and improved blood sugar control; 72.6% of patients who underwent the SADI-S had complete resolution of their type 2 diabetes.[44]

- Intragastric balloon

The IGB (**Fig. 6**) is a minimally invasive procedure in which a deflated balloon is inserted endoscopically into the stomach. The balloon is then inflated with saline which restricts the gut capacity, resulting in an increase in satiety and decrease in hunger, with less food consumption. The IGB is not a permanent procedure and must be removed after six months. Patients with a BMI above 30 are eligible for this procedure.[45,46]

Postoperative nutrition management

All bariatric surgeries require lifelong dietary compliance to ensure proper healing, as well as satisfactory and maintainable weight loss. One to two days postsurgery, the patient will consume only clear liquids. Graduation to the different foods in each post-surgical stage is customized and based on the individual patient and doctor's recommendations (see **Table 1**). New foods should be introduced one at a time, three days apart, to gauge for any adverse reactions.

Dietary compliance

Certain lifelong guidelines need to be followed to ensure weight loss, the integrity of the surgery, and adequate nutrient intake. Patients will eventually wean off protein supplements and consume the required amount of protein (60–80 grams/day) through the consumption of solid foods. Protein-rich foods need to be consumed first at each

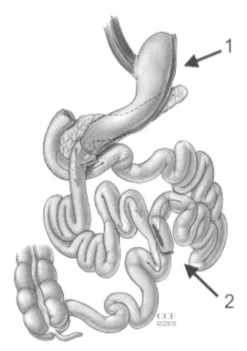

Fig. 4. Biliopancreatic diversion with duodenal switch. (1) Formation of gastric sleeve and its attachment to the area further down on small intestine where food is delivered (*orange arrows*). (2) Attachment of bypassed small intestine for provision of digestive juices (*green arrows*) needed for metabolism. (*From* the American Society for Bariatric and Metabolic Surgery[27];with permission.)

meal, vegetables second, and carbohydrates third (ideally healthy grains and/or fruits, not processed foods) (**Fig. 7**).

To reduce the risk of obstruction of the narrow opening between the stomach and small intestine, patients must eat slowly and chew thoroughly (to a pureed consistency) before swallowing. Proper hydration continues to be essential; 64 ounces of fluid is recommended daily (4 to 6 ounces/hour) to reduce the risk of constipation. Fluids must not be consumed with meals so nutrients in the food do not become diluted, and fullness is not experienced before ingestion of the meal. Therefore, fluid intake should be no less than 30 minutes before and after eating. As portion sizes are small, it is important to ensure the intake of nutrient dense foods; avoidance of calorically dense, processed foods is recommended. In addition, to avoid deficiencies, especially after malabsorptive procedures in which the body is unable to absorb sufficient nutrients, a daily multivitamin and mineral supplement is necessary.[48–51]

Food intolerances and nutrient deficiencies

Postsurgery, patients may experience food intolerances due to difficulty digesting certain foods. These can include red meat, pork, corn, popcorn, breads, raw vegetables, cooked fibrous/stringy vegetables, nuts, seeds, and beans; therefore, they should be consumed as individually tolerated.[53] Regarding inadequate levels of certain nutrients, 33–49% of patients present with iron-deficiency anemia within

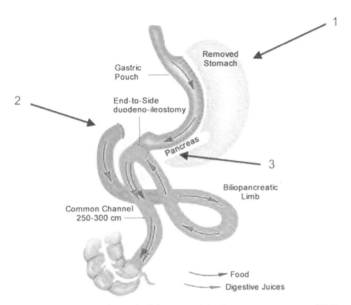

Fig. 5. Single anastamosis duodeno-ileal bypass with sleeve gastrectomy. (1) Formation of gastric sleeve. (2) Attachment of gastric sleeve to the ileal region of small intestine. (3) Bypassed area of the small intestine provides digestive juices for food entering the ileum. (*From* the American Society for Bariatric and Metabolic Surgery[27];with permission.)

2 years after surgery.[54] Macrocytic anemia, due to Vitamin B12 and folic acid deficiencies has been observed 5-years postsurgery in 19–35% and 9–39%, respectively.[55–57] Low levels of serum calcium and vitamin D are associated with a significant reduction in bone density (8–13%), a risk factor for osteoporosis.[58–60]

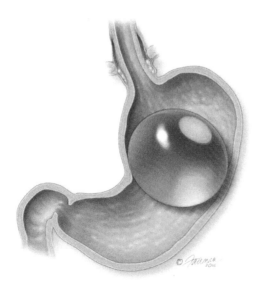

Fig. 6. Intragastric balloon insertion. ORBERA®, Apollo Endosurgery, Inc.[47]

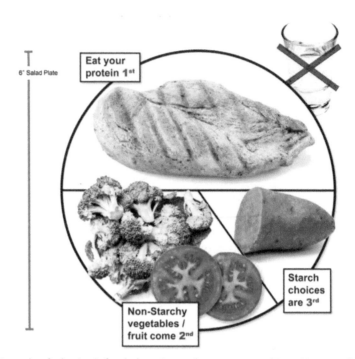

6" Salad Plate

Eat your protein 1st

Non-Starchy vegetables / fruit come 2nd

Starch choices are 3rd

Fig. 7. Example of a bariatric food plate, 6-months postsurgery. (*From* MetroHealth's Bariatric Plate for a Healthy Weight.[52])

The incidence of calcium and Vitamin D deficiencies are approximately 10% and 25–73%, respectively.[61,62] Clinical reports demonstrate low serum levels of the other fat-soluble vitamins (Vitamins A, K, and E) postsurgery, as well.[63] Deficiencies in the water-soluble vitamins, thiamine and vitamin C, can occur in up to 49% and 10–50%, respectively.[64–66] Among weight-loss surgery patients, the most insufficientmacronutrient in the diet is protein, with 7–21% of patients who underwent BPD-DS and 13% of patients who underwent GB, protein deficient after 2 years.[67] Possible etiologies for these nutrient deficiencies include hypochlorhydria, malabsorption attributed to the bypassing of the absorptive surfaces of the intestine, postoperative reduction in food intake due to restricted gastric capacity, changes in food preferences, and food intolerances.

Exercise

After bariatric surgery, regular physical activity is recommended as it is associated with decreased surgical complications and improvements in weight, body composition, and fitness.[68–70] There is substantial evidence to indicate that consistent physical activity is the most important predictor of long-term weight loss maintenance.[71] Exercise can also help improve bone density among patients with hypovitaminosis D and hypocalcemia.

Health Benefits

Bariatric surgery, in addition to the treatment of obesity, is highly effective in the management of type 2 diabetes, and other obesity-related diseases.[72–75] In a meta-analysis including a total of 22,094 patients, bariatric surgeries were associated with a total resolution in 76.8%, 61.7%, and 85.7% of patients with diabetes, hypertension, and obstructive sleep apnea, respectively, and an improvement in over 70% of patients with hyperlipidemia.[76]

FUTURE DIRECTIONS: EXPERIMENTAL WEIGHT LOSS SURGERIES
Gastric Plication Surgery

People with a BMI of 30–39.9 and an obesity-related disease may be candidates for this minimally invasive, reversible endoscopic procedure in which the stomach is folded inward and stitched in place, restricting capacity by 75%. Reported weight loss with this procedure is between 40 and 70% of excess weight among patients in the first year due to an increase in satiety and a reduction in food consumption.[87]

Endoluminal Liner

Also known as the duodenal–jejunal bypass sleeve, in this minimally invasive procedure, a flexible tube is inserted endoscopically, lining the first part of the small intestine. The tube acts as a barrier, delaying the absorption of food until further down the intestines, resulting in fewer calories yielded from food and an average loss of 19% of excess body weight.[88] This procedure significantly aids in the metabolic control of type 2 diabetes, as well.[87,89]

Endoscopic Sleeve Gastroplasty

During endoscopic sleeve gastroplasty (ESG), also known as the accordion procedure, 70–80% of the stomach is endoscopically sutured, creating a smaller stomach similar to LSG, but without removal of the remaining stomach. As this procedure is performed endoscopically vs laparoscopically, there are fewer surgical risks and post-surgical complications than with LSG. People with a BMI >30 who have been unsuccessful in maintaining weight loss with lifestyle modification alone or are looking for an alternative to traditional weight-loss surgeries may be candidates for ESG. Patients can expect to lose up to 20% of total body weight in the first 1 to 2 years.[90,91]

SUMMARY

National predictions estimate that by 2030, 50% of Americans will have obesity.[92] Bariatric surgeries are an option for people with an elevated BMI who have not been successful in keeping weight off through lifestyle changes, alone. Bariatric surgeries are not only associated with a loss of up to 80% excess body weight but the resolution of type 2 diabetes and other obesity-related health conditions, as well. Patients who undergo weight loss surgery are required to follow lifelong modifications in diet and behavior to maintain optimal weight loss and health benefits.

CLINICS CARE POINTS

- Patients with a BMI ≥30 may be candidates for bariatric surgery after trying other weight loss strategies without maintainable success.
- Weight loss surgeries work by restricting gut capacity, decreasing the absorption of nutrients and calories, or a combination of the two.
- Evaluate patient's needs to determine which surgery would be most suitable and explain the potential risks of each procedure.

- A lifetime commitment to dietary and behavioral modification is required postsurgery, including 60–80 grams of protein daily, and micronutrient supplements to reduce the risk of nutrient deficiencies, certain anemias and a reduction in bone density.
- Patients need to consume 64 ounces of fluids daily, no less than 30 minutes before or after a meal.

DISCLOSURE

The author has nothing to disclose.

REFERENCES

1. Hales CM, Fryar CD, Carroll MD, et al. Trends in obesity and severe obesity prevalence in US Youth and adults by sex and age, 2007-2008 to 2015-2016. JAMA 2018;319(16):1723–5.
2. Adult Obesity Facts. In: Center for disease control and prevention. Available at: https://www.cdc.gov/obesity/data/adult.html. Accessed January 4, 2022.
3. Kompaniyets L, Goodman AB, Belay B, et al. Body mass index and risk for COVID-19–related hospitalization, intensive care unit admission, invasive mechanical ventilation, and death — United States, March–December 2020. MMWR Morb Mortal Wkly Rep 2021;70:355–61.
4. Fryar CD, Carroll MD, Afful J. Prevalence of overweight, obesity, and severe obesity among adults aged 20 and over: United States, 1960–1962 through 2017–2018. In: National center for health statistics health E-stats. 2020. Available at: https://www.cdc.gov/nchs/data/hestat/obesity-adult-17-18/overweight-obesity-adults-H.pdf. Accessed January 15, 2022.
5. The health and economic cost of excess weight. In: Milken Institute. 2018. Available at: https://milkeninstitute.org/sites/default/files/reports-pdf/Mi-Americas-Obesity-Crisis-WEB_2.pdf. Accessed January 25, 2022.
6. Cawley J, Biener A, Meyerhoefer C, et al. Direct medical costs of obesity in the United States and the most populous states. J Manag Care Spec Pharm 2021; 27(3):354–66.
7. Gunnars K. 10 leading causes of weight gain and obesity. In: Healthline. 2022. Available at: https://www.healthline.com/nutrition/10-causes-of-weight-gain#TOC_TITLE_HDR_2. Accessed January 23, 2022.
8. Adamo KB, Ferraro ZM, Brett KE. Can we modify the intrauterine environment to halt the intergenerational cycle of obesity? Int J Environ Res Public Health 2012; 9(4):1263–307.
9. Kraschnewski JL, Boan J, Esposito J, et al. Long-term weight loss maintenance in the United States. Int J Obes 2010;34(11):1644–54.
10. Leibel RL, Rosenbaum M, Hirsch J. Changes in energy expenditure resulting from altered body weight. N Engl J Med 1995;332:621–8.
11. Ebbeling CB, Swain JF, Feldman HA, et al. Effects of dietary composition on energy expenditure during weight-loss maintenance. JAMA 2012;307:2627–34.
12. Martins C, Dutton GR, Hunter GR, et al. Revisiting the Compensatory Theory as an explanatory model for relapse in obesity management. Am J Clin Nutr 2020; 112(5):1170–9.
13. Prescription medications to treat overweight and obesity. In: National institute of diabetes and digestive and kidney health. 2021. Available at: https://www.niddk.nih.gov/health-information/weight-management/prescription-medications-treat-overweight-obesity#available. Accessed January 4, 2022.

14. Brown T, Avenell A, Edmunds LD, et al. Systematic review of long-term lifestyle interventions to prevent weight gain and morbidity in adults. Obes Rev 2009; 10(6):627–38.

15. Mann T, Tomiyama AJ, Westling E, et al. Medicare's search for effective obesity treatments: diets are not the answer. Am Psychol 2007;62(3):220–33.

16. Singh G, Krauthamer M, Bjalme-Evans M. Wegovy (semaglutide): a new weight loss drug for chronic weight management. J Investig Med 2022;70(1):5–13.

17. Avenell A, Broom J, Brown TJ, et al. Systematic review of the long-term effects and economic consequences of treatments for obesity and implications for health improvement. Health Technol Assess 2004;8(21):1–182, iii-iv.

18. Who is a candidate for bariatric surgery? In: American society for metabolic and bariatric surgery. Available at: https://asmbs.org/patients/who-is-a-candidate-for-bariatric-surgery. Accessed January 5, 2022.

19. Legner L. Disciplined diet before and after weight loss. In: OSF healthcare. 2021. Available at: https://www.osfhealthcare.org/blog/bariatric-surgery-diet/. Accessed January 4, 2022.

20. Types of gastric bypass. In: Stanford health care. Available at: https://stanfordhealthcare.org/medical-treatments/g/gastric-bypass-surgery/types.html. Accessed January 4, 2022.

21. Billeter AT, Fischer L, Wekerle AL, et al. Malabsorption as a Therapeutic Approach in Bariatric Surgery. Viszeralmedizin 2014;30(3):198–204.

22. Estimate of Bariatric Surgery Numbers, 2011-2019. In: American Society for metabolic and bariatric surgery. 2021. Available at: https://asmbs.org/resources/estimate-of-bariatric-surgery-numbers. Accessed January 5, 2022.

23. Nguyen NT, Goldman C, Rosenquist CJ, et al. Laparoscopic versus open gastric bypass: a randomized study of outcomes, quality of life, and costs. Ann Surg 2001;234:279–89.

24. Nguyen NT, Root J, Zainabadi K, et al. Accelerated growth of bariatric surgery with the introduction of minimally invasive surgery. Arch Surg 2005;140: 1198–202.

25. Puzziferri N, Austrheim-Smith IT, Wolfe BM, et al. Three-year follow-up of a prospective randomized trial comparing laparoscopic versus open gastric bypass. Ann Surg 2006;243:181–8.

26. Laparoscopic banding. In: MedlinePlus. 2020. Available at: https://medlineplus.gov/ency/article/007388.htm. Accessed January 22, 2022.

27. Bariatric surgery procedures. In: American society for metabolic and bariatric surgery. Available at: https://asmbs.org/patients/bariatric-surgery-procedures, 2021. Accessed January 22, 2022.

28. Falk V, Sheppard C, Kanji A, et al. The fate of laparoscopic adjustable gastric band removal. Can J Surg 2019;62(5):328–33.

29. Suter M, Calmes JM, Paroz A, et al. A 10-year experience with laparoscopic gastric banding for morbid obesity: high long-term complication and failure rates. Obes Surg 2006;16(7):829–35.

30. Gumbs AA, Gagner M, Dakin G, et al. Sleeve gastrectomy for morbid obesity. Obes Surg 2007;17:962–9.

31. Bohdjalian A, Langer FB, Shakeri-Leidenmuhler S, et al. Sleeve gastrectomy as sole and definitive bariatric procedure: 5-year results for weight loss and ghrelin. Obes Surg 2010;20:535–40.

32. Eisenberg D, Bellatorre A, Bellatorre N. Sleeve gastrectomy as a stand-alone bariatric operation for severe, morbid, and super obesity. JSLS 2013;17(1):63–7.

33. Stavros NMD, Vagenas, Konstantinos MD, et al. Weight loss, appetite suppression, and changes in fasting and postprandial ghrelin and peptide-YY levels after Roux-en-Y gastric bypass and sleeve gastrectomy. Ann Surg 2008;247(3):401–7.

34. Surgery for diabetes. In: American society for metabolic and bariatric surgery. 2021. Available at: https://asmbs.org/patients/surgery-for-diabetes. Accessed January 20, 2022.

35. Bariatric surgery procedures. In: American society for metabolic and bariatric surgery. 2022. Available at: https://asmbs.org/patients/bariatric-surgery-procedures#bypass. Accessed January 20, 2022.

36. Knop FK. Resolution of type 2 diabetes following gastric bypass surgery: involvement of gut-derived glucagon and glucagonotropic signalling? Diabetologia 2009;52:2270–6.

37. BPD-DS weight loss surgery. In: John hopkins medicine. Available at: https://www.hopkinsmedicine.org/health/treatment-tests-and-therapies/bpdds-weightloss-surgery. Accessed January 24, 2022.

38. Biliopancreatic diversion with duodenal switch. In: Mayo clinic. Available at: https://www.mayoclinic.org/tests-procedures/biliopancreatic-diversion-with-duodenal-switch/about/pac-20385180. Accessed January 20, 2022.

39. Kapeluto JE, Tchernof A, Masckauchan D, et al. Ten-year remission rates in insulin-treated type 2 diabetes after biliopancreatic diversion with duodenal switch. Surg Obes Relat Dis 2020;16(11):1701–12.

40. Ren CJ, Patterson E, Gagner M. Early results of laparoscopic biliopancreatic diversion with duodenal switch: a case series of 40 consecutive patients. Obes Surg 2000;10(6):514–23.

41. Sánchez-Pernaute A, Herrera MA, Pérez-Aguirre ME, et al. Single anastomosis duodeno-ileal bypass with sleeve gastrectomy (SADI-S). One to three-year follow-up. Obes Surg 2010;20(12):1720–6.

42. Sánchez-Pernaute A, Rubio MÁ, Cabrerizo L, et al. Single-anastomosis duodenoileal bypass with sleeve gastrectomy (SADI-S) for obese diabetic patients. Surg Obes Relat Dis 2015;11(5):1092–8.

43. Cottam D, Cottam S, Surve A. Single-Anastomosis Duodenal Ileostomy with Sleeve Gastrectomy "Continued Innovation of the Duodenal Switch. Surg Clin North Am 2021;101(2):189–98.

44. Spinos D, Skarentzos K, Esagian SM, et al. The Effectiveness of Single-Anastomosis Duodenoileal Bypass with Sleeve Gastrectomy/One Anastomosis Duodenal Switch (SADI-S/OADS): an Updated Systematic Review. Obes Surg 2021;31(4):1790–800.

45. Endoscopic weight loss program. In: John hopkins medicine. Available at: https://www.hopkinsmedicine.org/endoscopic-weight-loss-program/services/balloon.html. Accessed January 4, 2022.

46. Gastric balloons. In: Columbia, center for metabolic and weight loss surgery. Available at: https://columbiasurgery.org/conditions-and-treatments/gastric-balloons. Accessed January 15, 2022.

47. Obera™ gastric weight loss balloon. In: Moore metabolics. Available at: https://www.mooremetabolics.com/weight-loss/gastric-balloon/. Accessed February 7, 2022.

48. Gastric bypass diet: what to eat after surgery. In: Mayo clinic. Available at: https://www.mayoclinic.org/tests-procedures/gastric-bypass-surgery/in-depth/gastric-bypass-diet/art-20048472. Accessed January 10, 2022.

49. Dietary guidelines after bariatric surgery. In: UCSF health. Available at: https://www.ucsfhealth.org/education/dietary-guidelines-after-bariatric-surgery. Accessed January 15, 2022.

50. Adult bariatric surgery program. In: University of Michigan health system. Available at: https://www.med.umich.edu/bariatricsurgery/resources/Post-op-Diet-Sleeve.pdf. Accessed January 15, 2022.

51. Gastric bypass diet manual. In: Weight Management Center, Tower Health Medical Group. Available at: https://reading.towerhealth.org/app/files/public/451/gastricbypassdiet.pdf. Accessed January 21, 2022.

52. MetroHealth's bariatric plate for a healthy weight. In: The weight loss surgery and weight management center of methodist health. Available at: https://www.methodisthospital.org/documents/Bariatric-Plate.pdf. Accessed February 7, 2022.

53. Food Intolerance After Gastric Band Surgery. In: Health encyclopedia - university of rochester medical center. Available at: https://www.urmc.rochester.edu/encyclopedia/content.aspx?contenttypeid=134&contentid=104. Accessed January 26, 2022.

54. Iron deficiency anemia. In: American society of hematology. Available at: http://www.hematology.org/patients/blood-disorders/anemia/5263.aspx. Accessed March 8, 2022.

55. Blume CA, Boni CC, Casagrande DS, et al. Nutritional profile of patients before and after Roux-en-Y gastric bypass: 3-year follow-up. Obes Surg 2012;22:1676–85.

56. von Drygalski A, Andris DA, Nuttleman PR, et al. Anemia after bariatric surgery cannot be explained by iron deficiency alone: results of a large cohort study. Surg Obes Relat Dis 2011;7:151–6.

57. Shankar P, Boylan M, Sriram K. Micronutrient deficiencies after bariatric surgery. Nutrition 2010;26:1031–7.

58. Harper C, Pattinson AL, Fernando HA, et al. Effects of obesity treatments on bone mineral density, bone turnover and fracture risk in adults with overweight or obesity. Horm Mol Biol Clin Investig 2016;28:133–49.

59. Ko BJ, Myung SK, Cho KH, et al. Relationship between bariatric surgery and bone mineral density: a meta-analysis. Obes Surg 2016;26:1414–21.

60. Liu C, Wu D, Zhang JF, et al. Changes in bone metabolism in morbidly obese patients after bariatric surgery: a meta-analysis. Obes Surg 2016;26:91–7.

61. Shah M, Sharma A, Wermers RA, et al. Hypocalcemia after bariatric surgery: prevalence and associated risk factors. Obes Surg 2017;27:2905–11.

62. Chakhtoura MT, Nakhoul NN, Shawwa K, et al. Hypovitaminosis D in bariatric surgery: a systematic review of observational studies. Metabolism 2016;65:574–85.

63. Slater GH, Ren CJ, Siegel N, et al. Serum fat-soluble vitamin deficiency and abnormal calcium metabolism after malabsorptive bariatric surgery. J Gastrointest Surg 2004;8:48–55 [discussion: 54-55].

64. Milone M, Di Minno MN, Lupoli R, et al. Wernicke encephalopathy in subjects undergoing restrictive weight loss surgery: a systematic review of literature data. Eur Eat Disord Rev 2014;22:223–9.

65. Clements RH, Katasani VG, Palepu R, et al. Incidence of vitamin deficiency after laparoscopic Roux-en-Y gastric bypass in a university hospital setting. Am Surg 2006;72:1196–202 [discussion: 1203-1204].

66. Riess KP, Farnen JP, Lambert PJ, et al. Ascorbic acid deficiency in bariatric surgical population. Surg Obes Relat Dis 2009;5:81–6.

67. Faintuch J, Matsuda M, Cruz ME, et al. Severe protein-calorie malnutrition after bariatric procedures. Obes Surg 2004;14:175–81.
68. Egberts K, O'Brien PE. Optimising lifestyle factors to achieve weight loss in surgical patients. Surg Obes Relat Dis 2011;7(3):368.
69. Shah M, Snell PG, Rao S, et al. High-volume exercise program in obese bariatric surgery patients: a randomized, controlled trial. Obesity (Silver Spring) 2011; 19(9):1826–34.
70. McCullough PA, Gallagher MJ, Dejong AT, et al. Cardiorespiratory fitness and short-term complications after bariatric surgery. Chest 2006;130(2):517–25.
71. Donnelly JE, Blair SN, Jakicic JM, et al. American college of sports medicine american college of sports medicine position stand. appropriate physical activity intervention strategies for weight loss and prevention of weight regain for adults. Med Sci Sports Exerc 2009;41(2):459–71.
72. Singh AK, Singh R, Kota SK. Bariatric surgery and diabetes remission: who would have thought it? Indian J Endocrinol Metab 2015;19(5):563–76.
73. Pories WJ, Swanson MS, MacDonald KG, et al. Who would have thought it? An operation proves to be the most effective therapy for adult-onset diabetes mellitus. Ann Surg 1995;222:339–50.
74. Tsilingiris D, Koliaki C, Kokkinos A. Remission of type 2 diabetes mellitus after bariatric surgery: fact or fiction? Int J Environ Res Public Health 2019;16(17): 3171.
75. Schauer DP, Arterburn DE, Livingston EH, et al. Impact of bariatric surgery on life expectancy in severely obese patients with diabetes: a decision analysis. Ann Surg 2015;261(5):914–9.
76. Buchwald H, Avidor Y, Braunwald E, et al. Bariatric surgery: a systematic review and meta-analysis. JAMA 2004;292(14):1724–37.
77. Frezza EE. Laparoscopic vertical sleeve gastrectomy for morbid obesity. The future procedure of choice? Surg Today 2007;37(4):275–81.
78. Himpens J, Dapri G, Cadière GB. A prospective randomized study between laparoscopic gastric banding and laparoscopic isolated sleeve gastrectomy: results after 1 and 3 years. Obes Surg 2006;16(11):1450–6.
79. Gagner M, Buchwald JN. Comparison of laparoscopic sleeve gastrectomy leak rates in four staple-line reinforcement options: a systematic review. Surg Obes Relat Dis 2014;10(4):713–23.
80. Abou Rached A, Basile M, El Masri H. Gastric leaks post sleeve gastrectomy: review of its prevention and management. World J Gastroenterol 2014;20(38): 13904–10.
81. Pandolfino JE, Krishnamoorthy B, Lee TJ. Gastrointestinal complications of obesity surgery. MedGenMed 2004;6(2):15.
82. Pories WJ. Bariatric surgery: risks and rewards. J Clin Endocrinol Metab 2008; 93(11 Suppl 1):S89–96.
83. State of the Union. Weight Loss Surgery in 2022. In: Columbia, center for metabolic and weight loss surgery. Available at: https://columbiasurgery.org/news/state-union-weight-loss-surgery-2020. Accessed January 23, 2022.
84. Prachand VN, Davee RT, Alverdy JC. Duodenal switch provides superior weight loss in the super-obese (BMI > or =50 kg/m2) compared with gastric bypass. Ann Surg 2006;244(4):611–9.
85. MacLean LD, Rhode BM, Nohr CW. Late outcome of isolated gastric bypass. Ann Surg 2000;231(4):524–8.

86. Chang S, Stoll CRT, Song J, et al. The effectiveness and risks of bariatric surgery: an updated systematic review and meta-analysis, 2003-2012. JAMA Surg 2014; 149(3):275–87.
87. Jossart GH. Experimental weight loss surgery: the most 8 promising procedures. In: Bariatric surgery source. 2021. Available at: https://www.bariatric-surgery-source.com/experimental-weight-loss-surgery.html. Accessed January 23, 2022.
88. Tsuda S. Bariatric surgery: endoluminal techniques. In: Sages. Available at: https://www.sages.org/wiki/bariatric-surgery-endoluminal-techniques/. Accessed January 23, 2022.
89. Schouten R, Rijs CS, Bouvy ND, et al. A multicenter, randomized efficacy study of the EndoBarrier Gastrointestinal Liner for presurgical weight loss prior to bariatric surgery. Ann Surg 2010;251(2):236–43.
90. Wang JW, Chen CY. Current status of endoscopic sleeve gastroplasty: an opinion review. World J Gastroenterol 2020;26(11):1107–12.
91. Endoscopic sleeve gastroplasty. In: Mayo clinic. Available at: https://www.mayoclinic.org/tests-procedures/endoscopic-sleeve-gastroplasty/about/pac-20393958. Accessed January 24, 2022.
92. Ward ZJ, Bleich SN, Cradock AL, et al. Projected U.S. state-level prevalence of adult obesity and severe obesity. N Engl J Med 2019;381:2440–50.

Diet Strategies for the Patient with Chronic Kidney Disease

Susan Ettinger, PhD, RD, DABN

KEYWORDS

- Kidney disease • Gut microbiota • Ultraprocessed food • Acidosis • Bone disease
- Vascular calcification

KEY POINTS

- Consumption of ultraprocessed foods (UPF) with added sugars, fats, and additives and poor in fiber and nutrients is associated with metabolic diseases including chronic kidney disease (CKD). In contrast, whole unprocessed foods reduce the risk for CKD initiation and progression.
- Fiber-rich foods protect the gut barrier and prevent the translocation of pathogens and toxins into the blood. Consumption of fermentable fibers maintain populations of beneficial microbes that produce metabolites and nutrients absorbed by the host.
- Acid not excreted by the kidney enters the cells in exchange for cations such as potassium and magnesium. A diet rich in fruits and vegetables can lower the load of acid and retain cations in the cell, preventing dangerously high serum potassium levels.
- Simple sugars and refined starches are rapidly absorbed and can reach the kidney. If essential micronutrients are limited, both glucose and fructose are reabsorbed in the proximal tubule and can enter harmful metabolic pathways that produce uric acid and glycation products that subsequently damage the kidney.
- UPF contains multiple phosphate salts that approach 100% absorbability. A phosphate load triggers aberrant signals that increase bone resorption and cardiovascular damage. Phosphorous from whole foods, especially plant sources, is much less available. Plant sources also provide micronutrients that maintain bone structure and prevent vascular calcification.

INTRODUCTION

The global prevalence of diagnosed and undiagnosed adult diabetes has steadily increased during the past decades, from 151 million in 2000 to 451 million in 2017, with 693 million cases expected by 2045.[1] Approximately 40% of patients with either type I or II diabetes mellitus will develop diabetic kidney disease. Diabetes can result in

New York Institute of Technology, School of Health Professions, Northern Boulevard, P.O. Box 8000, Old Westbury, NY 11568-8000, USA
E-mail address: Ettingersusan64@gmail.com

Physician Assist Clin 7 (2022) 685–699
https://doi.org/10.1016/j.cpha.2022.06.002
2405-7991/22/© 2022 Elsevier Inc. All rights reserved.

Abbreviations	
UPF	ultraprocessed Foods
ESKD	end Stage Kidney Disease
SCFA	short Chain Fatty Acids
NAD	nicotine Adenine Diphosphate
NO	nitric Oxide
PRAL	potential Renal Acid Load
SSB	sweetened Beverages
PTH	parathyroid Hormone
VSMC	vascular Smooth Muscle Cells
MV	matrix Vesicles

multiple deleterious exposures that potentially damage the kidney, including hyperglycemia, hypertension, gut dysbiosis-derived toxins, drugs, and hypoxia. The pathogenesis of chronic kidney disease (CKD) includes mitochondrial dysfunction and apoptosis, overactivation of the renin-angiotensin system, inflammation, oxidative stress, podocyte loss, and fibrosis, all of which can exert collateral damage. Unchecked, these processes can interact and accelerate rapid progression to endstage kidney disease (ESKD). The National Kidney Foundation's Kidney Disease Outcomes Quality Initiative (KDOQI) Nutrition Guidelines provide comprehensive recommendations for the nutritional assessment and care of patients with CKD.[2] Detailed mechanisms linking pathogenesis and nutritional function are also found in the comprehensive text, Nutritional Management of Renal Disease.[3] Evidence that whole food can minimize kidney damage is also found in a recent text.[4] These resources support the use of selected patient-friendly diet strategies with the potential to slow progression to ESKD.

NUTRITIONAL STRATEGIES WITH POTENTIAL TO REDUCE RISK FOR CHRONIC KIDNEY DISEASE AND SLOW PROGRESSION TO END-STAGE KIDNEY DISEASE
1. Reduce Consumption of Ultraprocessed Foods and Increase Plant Foods

NOVA is a classification system that groups foods according to the physical, biological, and chemical processes used before the natural foods are consumed.[5] Ultraprocessed foods (UPF) have been described as industrial formulations of cheap energy and nutrient sources, usually denuded of fiber and laced with sugar, sodium, and other additives. UPF are energy dense, nutrient poor, and hyper-palatable, with long shelf lives and convenient to prepare and consume. Unfortunately, they are widely consumed. Data from the National Health and Nutrition Examination Survey (NHANES) 2000 to 2010 revealed that UPF made up more than 57% of the energy intake of the US diet. Added sugar represented 21% of the calories in UPF, compared with 2.4% in minimally processed food.[6] Using the NOVA metric, UPF consumption has been associated with significant declines in kidney function.[7,8] Further analysis of the NHANES data revealed that a diet high in UPF, although rich in added sugar and saturated fat, is poor in protein, fiber, vitamins A, C, D and E, as well as zinc, potassium, magnesium, and calcium (Ca).[9] It should be noted that other nutrients such as copper, folic acid, vitamins B6, B12, and K as well as bioactive components such as terpenes and polyphenols contained in whole foods were not measured.

However, plant-based diets, especially those rich in whole foods and low in UPF have been associated with reduction in the risk for kidney disease.[10] Adherence to a Mediterranean diet plan reduced renal function decline in prospective, multiethnic cohorts of healthy older adults.[11,12] The Dietary Approaches to Stop Hypertension

(DASH) diet was also effective in reducing kidney function decline in a multicenter cohort of African-American and Caucasian middle-aged subjects.[13] The 2020 KDOQI nutritional guidelines recommend the Mediterranean diet pattern to improve lipid profile and increased intake of fruits and vegetables to encourage weight loss, reduce blood pressure, and decrease the acid load.[14]

2. Consume Nutrients that Support Gut Barrier Function

The gut barrier is an integral part of innate host defense and includes both chemical and physical components. Antimicrobial proteins defend against diet-introduced bacteria while tight junctions between enterocytes and nutrient specific transport proteins assure that only essential molecules enter the blood. Enterocytes are protected from pathogens by 2 layers of viscous mucus and monitored by immune cells.[15] Commensal microbial populations protect the gut barrier by reducing growth of pathogenic bacteria and producing B vitamins (thiamin, riboflavin, niacin, folate, B12, B6, pantothenic acid) and vitamin K[16] and enhance the growth of microbial short chain fatty acid (SCFA) producers[17], thereby increasing nutrient availability to the host. Microbes produce retinoic acid (vitamin A) that provides epithelial defense and modulates vitamin A availability, preventing toxic levels.[18] Nicotine adenine diphosphate (NAD), necessary for mitochondrial biogenesis is maintained by cycling metabolites between host tissues and gut microbes.[19] Similarly, sodium nitrate contained in beets, celery, and other vegetables is converted by commensal microbes into nitric oxide (NO)[20], needed to dilate blood vessels, and sulfur donors in garlic and cruciferous vegetables are metabolized to beneficial hydrogen sulfide.[21]

A gut–kidney axis plays a major role in CKD progression.[22] Gut immune defenses and barrier functions are known to be impaired by exposure to uremic plasma,[23,24] suggesting that uremia causes dysbiosis. Microbes in the dysbiotic gut can produce harmful uremic toxins such as indoxyl sulfate and p-cresyl sulfate as well as triethylamine linked to cardiovascular disease. Reduced levels of beneficial bioactive metabolites including SCFA and essential nutrients have also been observed in the serum of patients with CKD. Dysbiosis results in activation of gut lymphoid tissue, proinflammatory mediator secretion and translocation of bacteria and toxins such as lipopolysaccharide through the permeable barrier. Bacterial translocation confirmed in the blood of nondialyzed patients with ESKD did not produce infection and was characterized as microinflammation.[25] Gut dysbiosis also increases production of reactive oxygen species (ROS) and is implicated in mitochondrial dysfunction.

Dietary strategies can cause or heal gut dysbiosis. Thus, a poor diet that causes gut dysbiosis can exacerbate kidney injury. Carbohydrate-consuming probiotics (microbes) are the primary producers of SCFA. They depend on prebiotics, especially fermentable carbohydrate fibers to provide their food. If dietary fibers are not provided, SCFA-producing microbes disappear, allowing overgrowth of pathogens capable of adapting their food supply to the carbohydrate-rich mucus, [26,27] thinning the protective mucosal barrier. Damaged enterocytes downregulate the production of antimicrobial proteins and tight junction linkages, increasing gut permeability and stimulating naïve T cells to differentiate into activated T cells rather than tolerant regulatory T cells.[28] Exogenous advanced glycation end-products (AGEs) produced by harsh food-processing methods[29] can be translocated across the gut and are implicated in the release of proinflammatory mediators, causing inflammation and fibrotic changes in the kidney.[30] UPF also contain emulsifiers (polysorbate 80) and additives (maltodextrose) that increase gut permeability by loosening tight junctions between enterocytes.[31,32]

In contrast, abundant research has demonstrated that prebiotics and bioactive compounds from plants, including highly colored fruits and vegetables modify gut bacteria; plant foods feed commensals and inhibit pathogens.[33–37] Mitochondrial function and NAD loss were ameliorated in mice with CKD and dysbiosis treated with SCFA-producing microbes.[38] Bioactive components provide a spectrum of anti-oxidant and anti-inflammatory actions that can reduce gut permeability to AGE complexes and other injurious metabolites.[26] Polyphenols and flavonoids have been shown to reduce the populations of microbial producers of uremic toxins and inhibit their metabolic activation.[39]

3. Reduce the Acid Load to Keep Potassium in the Cells

Metabolism of food produces anions (chlorine, phosphorous, sulfate), volatile organic acids and cations (sodium, potassium, calcium [Ca], magnesium [Mg]). When the diet provides more anions than cations, the kidney must excrete the acid as hydrogen ions (H^+) to maintain neutrality.[40] In the early stages of kidney failure, excess H^+ is buffered by bone and soft tissue in exchange for cations, potentiating CKD-associated bone and soft tissue abnormalities,[41] increased protein breakdown, inflammation and tubulointerstitial fibrosis.[42] The KDOQI recommendations suggest the use of sodium bicarbonate to maintain serum bicarbonate levels between 24 and 26 mMol/L.[2]

The potassium cation (K) is primarily intracellular and excreted by the kidney. Because it is critical for nerve transmission, patients with CKD with high-serum or low-serum K concentrations increase the risk for potentially fatal cardiac arrhythmias. In health, K intake is balanced by losses of K in the sweat, stool, and urine. Acid, also retained by the failing kidney, is taken into bone and tissue cells in exchange for K, exacerbating hyperkalemia. As the patient approaches ESKD, the gastrointestinal (GI) tract can adapt to increase K excretion across the gut mucosa by at least 3-fold. However, constipation is common in the patient with CKD due to multiple factors relating to the disease and treatment. Constipation reduces K excretion in the gut. The use of prebiotics and fiber-containing food is increasingly recommended,[43] not only to increase peristalsis and K excretion but also to modulate gut dysbiosis and increase lubricating mucus,[44] facilitating easier evacuation.

Dietary K restriction has been recommended to prevent or treat hyperkalemia in patients with CKD.[45] However, K derived from whole food has not been shown to significantly modify serum potassium levels,[46] possibly because the food matrix slows K absorption. More recent research suggests that diet modification to include cation producing foods such as fruits and vegetables, nuts, seeds, and legumes while reducing anion-producing foods such as grains, animal flesh, and hard cheeses[47] reduce the potential renal acid load (PRAL). The PRAL-lowering diet (**Fig. 1**) was shown to lower the acid load by 30% to 50%, the equivalent of supplementing 0.5 mEq/kg/d of sodium bicarbonate[48]; the typical Western diet with ∼ 15% to 17% of energy as protein, results in an average dietary acid load of approximately 1 mEq/kg/d. The DASH diet[13] reduces the acid load and slows the glomerular filtration rate (GFR) decline. Note that fats, oils, nuts, and seeds are relatively neutral and do not increase the acid load. Because fresh fruits and vegetables do not contain added sodium, diet modification of the acid load may be a better choice for the patient with CKD than sodium bicarbonate, which does increase the sodium load. As the kidney fails, choice of fiber-rich, but potassium poor, vegetables and sodium bicarbonate as toothpaste can be well tolerated and renoprotective, even in late-stage CKD.

4, Avoid Simple Sugar/Refined Starch and Improve Energy Production

Sugar sweetened beverages (SSB) increase the risk for chronic disease.[49] Meta-analysis of 17 cohort studies revealed that an increase of 1 SSB/d increased the risk for type II diabetes, even after correcting for adiposity.[50] SSB intake also

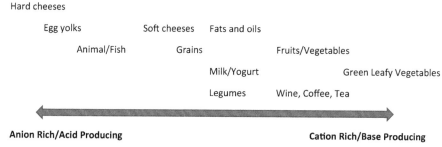

Hard cheeses

Egg yolks   Soft cheeses   Fats and oils

Animal/Fish   Grains   Fruits/Vegetables

Milk/Yogurt   Green Leafy Vegetables

Legumes   Wine, Coffee, Tea

Anion Rich/Acid Producing   **Cation Rich/Base Producing**

Fig. 1. The PRAL diet. A plant-based diet rich in fruits and vegetables contains more cations (sodium, potassium, calcium, magnesium) that can balance the excess H^+ that the failing kidney cannot excrete. Note that fats, oils, nuts, and seeds are relatively neutral and do not increase the acid load. Because fresh fruits and vegetables do not contain added sodium, diet modification of the acid load may be a better choice for the CKD patient than sodium bicarbonate, which does provide sodium. (*Adapted from* Scialla JJ, Anderson CA. Dietary acid load: a novel nutritional target in chronic kidney disease?. *Adv Chronic Kidney Dis.* 2013;20(2):141-149.)

increased the risk for CKD in a population of community-based black American subjects.[51] The fructose:glucose ratio in SSB is greater than 1.1; the ratio in apple juice is 2:1 or greater.[52] Elevated CKD risk from SSB has been linked to rapid fructose absorption, especially when SSB are consumed without food matrix present. The enterocyte metabolizes the small amounts of fructose in whole foods to glucose and organic acids.[53] However, a high-fructose load can escape the gut and enter the systemic circulation.[54] In contrast to glucose, fructose metabolism is not regulated, thus high-fructose loads are metabolized in the liver to lipids and uric acid.[55] Some of the high-fructose load reaches the kidney where it is taken up by the glucose receptors (GLUT 5) in the proximal convoluted tubule (PCT). Fructose metabolism requires the high energy molecule, adenosine triphosphate (ATP), thus a high fructose load not only limits the amount of ATP for the high energy demands of the PCT[56] but uric acid produced stimulates proinflammatory mediators and inhibits endothelial NO synthase, reducing NO availability and triggering vasoconstriction and tubulointerstitial fibrosis. Uric acid also stimulates the expression of adhesion molecules, activates inflammatory macrophages, and transforms fibroblasts into myofibroblasts.[57]

The glucose polymer in refined starch is rapidly digested and the glucose absorbed, raising blood glucose levels. Glucose is filtered by the kidney and resorbed in the PCT where it can enter several metabolic pathways (**Fig. 2**). Some of these pathways produce harmful metabolites. The polyol pathway produces endogenous fructose that is further metabolized to potentially toxic uric acid, whereas nonenzymatic glycation produces AGEs that can cross-link matrices, stiffen arteries and stimulate proinflammatory signals that lead to oxidative stress and fibrosis.[58] Fructose has been shown to be 7-fold to 10-fold better than other sugars as a substrate for AGE.[59] In the failing kidney, when the mitochondria become dysfunctional, metabolites such as pyruvate accumulate in the cytoplasm.[60] It has been suggested that endogenous fructose acts as a metabolic switch to bypass the mitochondria and stimulate glycolysis, thereby supplying intermediates to potentially inflammatory pathways in a manner similar to the Warburg effect.[61]

Some pathways are beneficial. The pentose phosphate shunt (PPS) consumes glucose and produces ribose and nicotinamide adenine dinucleotide phosphate (NADPH), an essential electron donor required for the reduction of oxidized glutathione.

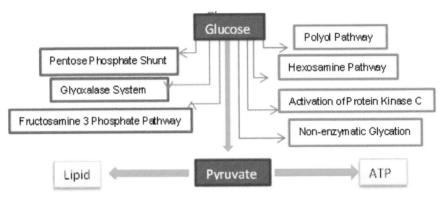

Fig. 2. Glucose pathways. In addition to the glycolytic pathway (center), glucose can enter several other pathways. "Harmful" pathways (*blue*) contribute to oxidative metabolites and diabetic complications. "Protective" metabolic pathways (*red*) convert glucose into harmless or useful metabolites. The pentose phosphate shunt (PPS) is especially useful because it produces both ribose substrate for nucleotide biosynthesis and NADPH required for antioxidant protection and for oxygen-dependent killing by phagocytic cells. Thiamin is required as cofactor for *transketolase* in PPP. (*Figure adapted from* Pácal L, Tomandl J, Svojanovsky J, et al. Role of thiamine status and genetic variability in transketolase and other pentose phosphate cycle enzymes in the progression of diabetic nephropathy. *Nephrol Dial Transplant.* 2011;26(4):1229-1236.)

Glutathione antioxidant defense is compromised in patients with CKD.[62] Thiamin is a required cofactor for *transketolase*, a limiting enzyme for the PPS. Thiamin is also required for *pyruvate dehydrogenase*, the complex that converts pyruvate to acetyl coenzyme A, allowing pyruvate entrance into the mitochondrial citric acid cycle and ATP synthesis. Thus, thiamin is critical for reducing glucose flux into harmful pathways.

Thiamin is found in meat, especially pork, fish, the seed coat of grains, seeds, legumes, and nuts. Flour and other staple foods are fortified with thiamin.[63] Despite its availability in foods, thiamin deficiency is common but often overlooked.[64] Serum thiamin levels were 75% lower in diabetics than in normal controls.[65] Thiamin depletion in patients with CKD can be due to glucose-induced downregulation of the PCT thiamin transporters,[66] as well as poor diet intake, inflammation, alcohol consumption, high carbohydrate intake, and loop diuretic-induced loss in the urine.[67] The uremic toxin, oxythiamine, formed by exposing thiamin-containing foods to acid and high heat, can be absorbed through a permeable gut, and has been implicated in thiamin dysfunction.[68] Thiamin conversion to thiamin pyrophosphate, its active cofactor, requires a Mg cofactor and ATP.[69] Thus, concomitant Mg deficiency can also inhibit thiamin activity. Supplementation with 100 mg thiamin OK has been recommended for at-risk patients with CKD.[67] Appropriate assessment methodologies and clinical recommendations for micronutrients are comprehensively discussed by Kopple and colleagues.[70]

Mg is especially important in slowing progression to ESKD.[71] Mg downregulates inflammation by regulating inflammatory cascades such as nuclear factor kappa beta (NFkβ) and tumor necrosis factor (TNF), inhibits differentiation of activated inflammatory cells, and inhibits production of inflammatory cytokines. These actions reduce inflammation and ROS in the kidney. Mg also reduces the activity of caspase and prevents cell death through apoptosis. Mg is thought to regulate the Ca transporter and a membrane protein, Klotho, involved in bone metabolism (see later discussion). It is also known to reduce mitochondrial dysfunction by inhibiting L-type Ca channels and reducing the rate of renal fibrosis.

Mg is the central atom in chlorophyll, thus green leafy vegetables are rich dietary Mg sources. Other plant sources include seeds, nuts, grains, legumes, and dark chocolate. Although the patient with CKD is often told to avoid these foods because they also contain potassium, plant-based foods provide a low acid load and are beneficial to both potassium status and acid–base balance.[72] Mg is poorly absorbed (about 30%) and several drugs including loop and thiazide diuretics, chemotherapeutic agents and proton pump inhibitors are associated with Mg loss.

Mitochondrial dysfunction in CKD is exacerbated by ROS and by downregulation of protective cascades such as nuclear factor-erythroid factor 2 related factor 2 (Nrf2), a transcription factor that regulates expression of more than 1000 protective genes.[73,74] Nrf2 is activated by bioactive components in the diet and by microbial metabolites. Mitochondrial dysfunction and DNA damage are also seen when folate and vitamins B6 and B12 are limiting. These nutrients regulate the methionine and transsulfuration cycles that maintain homocysteine (Hcy), a highly reactive oxidant, at normal levels (**Fig. 3**). Hyperglycemia blocks the transulfuration pathway and allows Hcy to accumulate.[75,76] Hcy oxidizes proteins, impairs nitric oxide production, and lead to endothelial dysfunction. Preliminary evidence suggests that dietary polyphenols, including sulforaphane (broccoli) and curcumin (turmeric) as well as purple fruits and vegetables (anthocyanin) stimulate mitochondria biogenesis in vitro, can be effective as adjuvant therapy for the patient with CKD.[77]

5. Maintain Bone and Vessel Integrity

Abnormal bone mineral homeostasis in CKD fosters the development of renal osteodystrophy and vascular calcification. Ca, phosphate (P), Mg, and vitamin D (Vit D) and

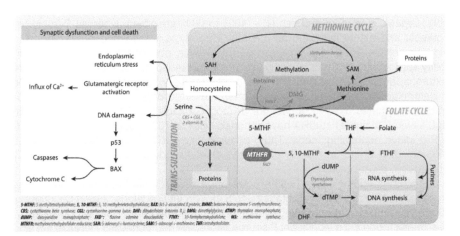

Fig. 3. Methionine and Transsulfuration Pathways. Methionine (Met), an essential amino acid for protein biosynthesis, is combined with adenosine and ATP to form S-adenosylmethionine (SAM), a universal methyl donor. Demethylated S-adenosyl homocysteine is recycled to homocysteine and remethylated by 5-methyl tetrahydrofolate (5-MTHF) and *methionine synthase* using a vitamin B12 cofactor. Hcy is also metabolized by the transsulfuration pathway. B6-dependant enzymes convert Hcy to cysteine (Cys) required for protein biosynthesis and also the rate limiting substrate for the synthesis of glutathione, a major endogenous antioxidant and for the gasotransmitter hydrogen sulfide (not shown). Inhibition of either cycle by nutrient deficiency results in a highly reactive Hcy lactone that activates DNA damage and cell death. (tGuillaume Pelletier, CC BY-SA 3.0 <https:// creativecommons.org/licenses/by-sa/3.0>, via Wikimedia Commons)

vitamin K (Vit K) are essential for bone crystal maintenance and for the prevention of soft tissue calcification. Regulation of serum Ca by parathyroid hormone and active Vit D (1-25D) and the phosphaturic action of fibroblast growth factor 23 (FGF23) have been described.[78,79] Current understanding of the integrated regulation of these nutrients in bone mineral homeostasis is discussed in Kopple and colleagues.[4,80–82]

Briefly, following absorption, serum P indirectly stimulates FGF23 production by bone.[82] FGF23 secretion is also stimulated by parathyroid hormone (PTH), hypercalcemia and 1-25D. FGF23 binds its coreceptor, Klotho, on the PCT membrane and downregulates P transporters in the kidney tubules, facilitating P excretion. Klotho binding also downregulates 1-25 D biosynthesis, reducing GI absorption of both Ca and P. If the serum Ca reduces too low, PTH is secreted, activating 1-25D production and facilitating Ca and P release from bone, Ca absorption in the gut and net Ca resorption in the kidney. Together, these actions return serum Ca to its normal range.

As the kidney fails, less Klotho is available at the PCT for FGF-23 signaling; without Klotho binding, the kidney excretes less P in the urine. Serum P increases, further stimulating secretion of FGF23. The parathyroid gland also requires Klotho to bind FGF23. FGF23-Klotho binding suppresses PTH secretion when Ca is normal, elevates PTH when serum Ca is low, and suppresses parathyroid gland proliferation. Klotho loss and elevated FGF23 in CKD precipitate secondary parathyroid hyperplasia; more gland cells secrete more PTH that increases serum Ca levels due to bone resorption.[83] Klotho is not required for FGF23 to bind its recepter (FGFR4) in the heart. Thus, elevated FGF23 levels in CKD stimulate ventricular hypertrophy[84] and also stimulate hepatic secretion of proinflammatory cytokines, contributing to inflammation in the patient with CKD.[82]

As the patient reaches CKD stage 3, dietary modulation of phosphorous intake becomes a mainstay of diet therapy.[85] Dietary phosphorous bioavailability is highly variable. Organic P in meat and fish is ~ 40% to 60% absorbed, whereas P in grains, legumes, and plants is bound as phytate, a poorly absorbed phosphate complex, allowing only ~ 10% to 30% absorption. However, phosphate salts with bioavailability approaching 100% are widely used in processed foods as additives to enhance texture, appearance, and shelf life. The exact intake of phosphate salts is impossible to determine because P-additives are often not listed on the label and many food-grade phosphates used in agriculture or food packaging are not measured.[86,87] In fact, several analytical studies have reported 25% to 70% underrepresentation of P in P-additive-containing foods. Thus, patients with CKD are well advised to avoid UPF including bread and highly processed animal products and consume a largely whole food, plant-based diet.[88]

Ca recommendations for a healthy adult range from 1000 to 1500 mg/d, depending on age.[89] In patients with CKD stages 3 to 5, not on Vit D analogs, a total Ca intake of 800 to 1000 mg/d, is recommended.[2] Ca is well absorbed from dairy products; however, these foods are a significant P source. Moreover, hard cheeses increase the acid load and can promote bone buffering and Ca loss. Ca is also found in legumes, seeds, and green leafy vegetables. Most phosphorous in these foods is bound as phytate and is poorly absorbed. Although these foods contain potassium, experimental and epidemiologic evidence suggests that dietary potassium from whole foods is beneficial, in contrast to potassium salts and additives. Adequate potassium benefits the kidney, reduces blood pressure, improves sodium excretion, and reduces the risk for cardiovascular disease.[90]

Risk for soft tissue calcification was formerly predicted when an ionic Ca x P product threshold was exceeded in CKD stage 3 to 5 patients.[91] It is now known that serum phosphate is taken into vascular smooth muscle cells (VSMC) by sodium-dependent phosphate cotransporters and the VSMC is stimulated to undergo osteochondrogenic phenotypic change and to secrete extracellular collagen matrix. High Ca due to PTH hypersecretion also enters the VSMC. VSMC compensate for high intracellular Ca/P concentrations by forming protected matrix vesicles (MVs) that allow $CaHPO_4$ crystals to be safely formed. MV induce expressions of genes that promote VSMC transdifferentiation to an osteoblast-like cell that secretes hydroxyapatite crystals $[Ca_5(PO_4)_3(OH)]$ onto the newly formed collagen matrix; crystals subsequently exchange or adsorb ions onto their surface.[92]. This process results in vascular calcification (VC) and its complications.

Low serum Mg has been inversely associated withVC, cardiovascular events, and mortality in patients with CKD.[93] Mg limits VC by forming smaller, Mg-substituted (whitlockite) crystals that inhibit the transformation of amorphous Ca/P to mature hydroxyapatite. Mg also antagonizes Ca channels, reducing Ca uptake into the cells. Finally, Mg enters the cell via its receptor and neutralizes the phosphate-induced inhibition of the calcification inhibitors such as vitamin K-dependent matrix gla protein (MGP) and bone matrix protein 7 (BMP7). Mg also downregulates genes that promote VSMC conversion to an osteoblast phenotype.[94]

VC and its devastating exacerbation, calciphylaxis, have been linked to inactivation of crystallization inhibitors.[95] When activated (carboxylated) by Vit K, MGP binds Ca and inhibits damage to the vascular elastic fibers and VC.[96] When dietary Vit K is limiting or when Vit K recycling is inhibited by drugs, MGPs in the VSMC remain uncarboxylated and inactive.[97] Vit K found in green leafy vegetables, vegetable oils, nuts, and legumes is metabolized to its active form by gut bacteria; active Vit K is also found in fermented vegetables and cheeses. Vit K deficiency has been reported even in patients with early CKD due to drugs (eg, Warfarin) and antibiotics as well as restricted diet and gut dysbiosis.

Vit K also maintains bone integrity by carboxylating osteocalcin, involved in bone matrix synthesis and regulation of mineral maturation in the bone. Inhibition of 1-25D activation in CKD leads to reduced synthesis of OC in osteoblasts.[98] Inadequate Vit K status has been positively associated with the circulating concentration of undercarboxylated osteocalcin and to the frequency of fractures in hemodialysis patients. Low levels of carboxylated MGP in bone lead to increased osteoclast activity and bone resorption.

SUMMARY

Two millennia ago, Hippocrates understood the importance of diet and lifestyle in preventing and ameliorating disease.[99] After decades of restricting protein, potassium, and phosphorous and offering the patient with CKD on dialysis lemon drop candy to reduce their thirst, the value of a whole food diet is gaining appreciation.[74] This review of the current literature has provided several strategies that seem most useful as a first approximation of diet therapy for the patient with CKD. However, the diet for the kidney patient is complex, and these patients are best advised by a Registered Dietitian Nutritionist who specializes in this area and is part of the health-care team.

CLINICS CARE POINTS

- Restrict ultraprocessed food containing chemical additives as much as possible.
- Encourage home cooking methods because commercially prepared foods tend to be high in sodium, sugars, and additives.
- Restrict SSB due to their association with an increased risk for diabetes and CKD.

- Encourage a whole food disuch as a Mediterranean or DASH type diet that is moderate in animal proteins and rich in plant sources such as legumes, nuts, whole grains, vegetables, and fruits.
- Recommene consumption of prebiotics and fiber-containing foods .
- As the patient reaches CKD stage 3, dietary modulation of phosphorous intake becomes a mainstay of diet therapy.
- In patients with CKD stages 3 to 5, not on Vit D analogs, a total Ca intake of 800 to 1000 mg/ d is recommended.
- Refer to the 2020 National Kidney Foundation's KDOQI guideline 14 for appropriate protein and energy requirements for the patient CKD stage.

DISCLOSURE

The author has nothing to disclose.

REFERENCES

1. Cho NH, Shaw JE, Karuranga S, et al. IDF Diabetes Atlas: Global estimates of diabetes prevalence for 2017 and projections for 2045. Diabetes Res Clin Pract 2018;138:271–81.
2. Ikizler TA, Cuppari L. Chapter 1 - The KDOQI Clinical Practice Guidelines for Nutrition in CKD: 2020 update. In: Kopple JD, Massry SG, Kalantar-Zadeh K, et al, editors. Nutritional management of renal disease. 4th edition. Academic Press; 2022. p. 3–7.
3. Kopple JD. Contents. In: Kopple JD, Massry SG, Kalantar-Zadeh K, et al, editors. Nutritional management of renal disease. 4th edition. Academic Press; 2021. vii-xv.
4. Ettinger S. Chapter 7 - Diabetic Nephropathy, Chronic Kidney Disease. In: Ettinger S, editor. Nutritional pathophysiology of obesity and its comorbidities. Academic Press; 2017. p. 161–89.
5. Monteiro CA, Cannon G, Moubarac JC, et al. The UN Decade of Nutrition, the NOVA food classification and the trouble with ultra-processing. Public Health Nutr 2018;21(1):5–17.
6. Martínez Steele E, Baraldi LG, Louzada MLdC, et al. Ultra-processed foods and added sugars in the US diet: evidence from a nationally representative cross-sectional study. BMJ Open 2016;6(3):e009892.
7. Cai Q, Duan M, Dekker LH, et al. FC 081ultra-processed food consumption and risk of incident chronic kidney disease: the lifelines cohort. Nephrol Dial Transplant 2021;36(Supplement_1):FC081.
8. Rey-García J, Donat-Vargas C, Sandoval-Insausti H, et al. Ultra-processed food consumption is associated with renal function decline in older adults: a prospective cohort study. Nutrients 2021;13(2).
9. Martínez Steele E, Popkin BM, Swinburn B, et al. The share of ultra-processed foods and the overall nutritional quality of diets in the US: evidence from a nationally representative cross-sectional study. Popul Health Metrics 2017;15(1):6.
10. Joshi S, McMacken M, Kalantar-Zadeh K. Plant-based diets for kidney disease: a guide for clinicians. Am J Kidney Dis 2021;77(2):287–96.
11. Khatri M, Moon YP, Scarmeas N, et al. The association between a Mediterranean-style diet and kidney function in the Northern Manhattan Study cohort. Clin J Am Soc Nephrol 2014;9(11):1868–75.

12. Bayán-Bravo A, Banegas JR, Donat-Vargas C, et al. The mediterranean diet protects renal function in older adults: a prospective cohort study. Nutrients 2022;14(3).

13. Rebholz CM, Crews DC, Grams ME, et al. DASH (dietary approaches to stop hypertension) diet and risk of subsequent kidney disease. Am J Kidney Dis 2016; 68(6):853–61.

14. Ikizler TA, Burrowes JD, Byham-Gray LD, et al. KDOQI Clinical Practice Guideline for Nutrition in CKD: 2020 Update. Am J Kidney Dis 2020;76(3, Supplement 1): S1–107.

15. Vaziri ND, Goshtasbi N, Yuan J, et al. Uremic Plasma Impairs Barrier Function and Depletes the Tight Junction Protein Constituents of Intestinal Epithelium. Am J Nephrol 2012;36(5):438–43.

16. LeBlanc JG, Milani C, de Giori GS, et al. Bacteria as vitamin suppliers to their host: a gut microbiota perspective. Curr Opin Biotechnol 2013;24(2):160–8.

17. Soto-Martin EC, Warnke I, Farquharson FM, et al. Vitamin Biosynthesis by Human Gut Butyrate-Producing Bacteria and Cross-Feeding in Synthetic Microbial Communities. mBio 2020;11(4).

18. Woo V, Eshleman EM, Hashimoto-Hill S, et al. Commensal segmented filamentous bacteria-derived retinoic acid primes host defense to intestinal infection. Cell Host & Microbe 2021;29(12):1744–56.e1745.

19. Chellappa K, McReynolds MR, Lu W, et al. NAD precursors cycle between host tissues and the gut microbiome. bioRxiv 2021.

20. Parthasarathy DK, Bryan NS. Sodium nitrite: The "cure" for nitric oxide insufficiency. Meat Sci 2012;92(3):274–9.

21. Blachier F, Andriamihaja M, Larraufie P, et al. Production of hydrogen sulfide by the intestinal microbiota and epithelial cells and consequences for the colonic and rectal mucosa. Am J Physiology-Gastrointestinal Liver Physiol 2021;320(2): G125–35.

22. Cao C, Zhu H, Yao Y, et al. Gut dysbiosis and kidney diseases. Front Med (Lausanne) 2022;9:829349.

23. Anders HJ, Andersen K, Stecher B. The intestinal microbiota, a leaky gut, and abnormal immunity in kidney disease. Kidney Int 2013;83(6):1010–6.

24. Betjes MG. Uremia-associated ageing of the thymus and adaptive immune responses. Toxins 2020;12(4):224.

25. Wang F, Jiang H, Shi K, et al. Gut bacterial translocation is associated with microinflammation in end-stage renal disease patients. Nephrology (Carlton). 2012; 17(8):733–8.

26. Martel J, Chang S-H, Ko Y-F, et al. Gut barrier disruption and chronic disease. Trends Endocrinol Metab 2022;33(4):247–65.

27. Desai Mahesh S, Seekatz Anna M, Koropatkin Nicole M, et al. A dietary fiber-deprived gut microbiota degrades the colonic mucus barrier and enhances pathogen susceptibility. Cell 2016;167(5):1339–53.e1321.

28. Allaire JM, Crowley SM, Law HT, et al. The intestinal epithelium: central coordinator of mucosal immunity. Trends Immunology 2018;39(9):677–96.

29. Bettiga A, Fiorio F, Di Marco F, et al. The Modern Western Diet Rich in Advanced Glycation End-Products (AGEs): an overview of its impact on obesity and early progression of renal pathology. Nutrients 2019;11(8):1748.

30. Rabbani N, Thornalley PJ. Advanced glycation end products in the pathogenesis of chronic kidney disease. Kidney Int 2018;93(4):803–13.

31. Khuda SE, Nguyen AV, Sharma GM, et al. Effects of emulsifiers on an in vitro model of intestinal epithelial tight junctions and the transport of food allergens. Mol Nutr Food Res 2022;66(4):2100576.

32. Laudisi F, Di Fusco D, Dinallo V, et al. The food additive maltodextrin promotes endoplasmic reticulum stress–driven mucus depletion and exacerbates intestinal inflammation. Cell Mol Gastroenterol Hepatol 2019;7(2):457–73.

33. Cai T-T, Ye X-L, Li R-R, et al. Resveratrol modulates the gut microbiota and inflammation to protect against diabetic nephropathy in mice. Front Pharmacol 2020; 11:1–13.

34. Hsu C-N, Hou C-Y, Chang C-I, et al. Resveratrol butyrate ester protects adenine-treated rats against hypertension and kidney disease by regulating the gut–kidney axis. Antioxidants 2021;11(1):83.

35. Yao M, Fei Y, Zhang S, et al. Gut microbiota composition in relation to the metabolism of oral administrated resveratrol. Nutrients 2022;14(5):1013.

36. Bao N, Chen F, Dai D. The regulation of host intestinal microbiota by polyphenols in the development and prevention of chronic kidney disease. Front Immunol 2020;10.

37. Mu J, Xu J, Wang L, et al. Anti-inflammatory effects of purple sweet potato anthocyanin extract in DSS-induced colitis: modulation of commensal bacteria and attenuated bacterial intestinal infection. Food Funct 2021;12(22):11503–14.

38. Yu SM-W, He JC. Happy gut, happy kidneys? Restoration of gut microbiome ameliorates acute and chronic kidney disease. Cell Metab 2021;33(10):1901–3.

39. Singhal S, Rani V. Study to explore plant-derived trimethylamine lyase enzyme inhibitors to address gut dysbiosis. Appl Biochem Biotechnol 2022;194(1):99–123.

40. Scialla JJ, Anderson CAM. Dietary acid load: a novel nutritional target in chronic kidney disease? Adv Chronic Kidney Dis 2013;20(2):141–9.

41. Melamed ML, Raphael KL. Metabolic acidosis in CKD: a review of recent findings. Kidney Med 2021;3(2):267–77.

42. Wesson DE, Buysse JM, Bushinsky DA. Mechanisms of metabolic acidosis-induced kidney injury in chronic kidney disease. J Am Soc Nephrol 2020;31(3):469–82.

43. Su G, Qin X, Yang C, et al. Fiber intake and health in people with chronic kidney disease. Clin Kidney J 2021;15(2):213–25.

44. Ikee R, Yano K, Tsuru T. Constipation in chronic kidney disease: it is time to reconsider. Ren Replace Ther 2019;5(1):51.

45. St-Jules DE, Goldfarb DS, Sevick MA. Nutrient non-equivalence: does restricting high-potassium plant foods help to prevent hyperkalemia in hemodialysis patients? J Ren Nutr 2016;26(5):282–7.

46. St-Jules DE, Shah A. Chapter 21 - Management of potassium in chronic kidney disease and acute kidney injury. In: Kopple JD, Massry SG, Kalantar-Zadeh K, et al, editors. Nutritional management of renal disease. 4th edition. Academic Press; 2022. p. 329–43.

47. Remer T, Manz F. Potential renal acid load of foods and its influence on urine pH. J Am Diet Assoc 1995;95(7):791–7.

48. Goraya N, Raphael KL, Wesson DE. Chapter 19 - Alkalization to retard progression of chronic kidney disease. In: Kopple JD, Massry SG, Kalantar-Zadeh K, et al, editors. Nutritional management of renal disease. 4th edition. Academic Press; 2022. p. 297–309.

49. Malik VS, Hu FB. The role of sugar-sweetened beverages in the global epidemics of obesity and chronic diseases. Nat Rev Endocrinol 2022;18(4):205–18.

50. Imamura F, O'Connor L, Ye Z, et al. Consumption of sugar sweetened beverages, artificially sweetened beverages, and fruit juice and incidence of type 2 diabetes: systematic review, meta-analysis, and estimation of population attributable fraction. BMJ (Clinical research ed) 2015;351:h3576.
51. Rebholz CM, Young BA, Katz R, et al. Patterns of beverages consumed and risk of incident kidney disease. Clin J Am Soc Nephrol 2019;14(1):49–56.
52. DeChristopher LR, Tucker KL. Excess free fructose, apple juice, high fructose corn syrup and childhood asthma risk – the National Children's Study. Nutr J 2020;19(1):60.
53. Jang C, Wada S, Yang S, et al. The small intestine shields the liver from fructose-induced steatosis. Nat Metab 2020;2(7):586–93.
54. Francey C, Cros J, Rosset R, et al. The extra-splanchnic fructose escape after ingestion of a fructose-glucose drink: An exploratory study in healthy humans using a dual fructose isotope method. Clin Nutr ESPEN 2019;29:125–32.
55. Mastrocola R, Ferrocino I, Liberto E, et al. Fructose liquid and solid formulations differently affect gut integrity, microbiota composition and related liver toxicity: a comparative in vivo study. J Nutr Biochem 2018;55:185–99.
56. Milutinović DV, Brkljačić J, Teofilović A, et al. Chronic stress potentiates high fructose–induced lipogenesis in rat liver and kidney. Mol Nutr Food Res 2020; 64(13):1901141.
57. Nakagawa T, Kang D-H. Fructose in the kidney: from physiology to pathology. Kidney Res Clin Pract 2021;40(4):527–41.
58. Ito M, Gurumani MZ, Merscher S, et al. Glucose- and non-glucose-induced mitochondrial dysfunction in diabetic kidney disease. Biomolecules 2022;12(3).
59. Aragno M, Mastrocola R. Dietary sugars and endogenous formation of advanced glycation endproducts: emerging mechanisms of disease. Nutrients 2017; 9(4):385.
60. Schaub JA, Venkatachalam MA, Weinberg JM. Proximal tubular oxidative metabolism in acute kidney injury and the transition to CKD. Kidney360. 2021;2(2): 355–64.
61. Nakagawa T, Sanchez-Lozada LG, Andres-Hernando A, et al. Endogenous fructose metabolism could explain the warburg effect and the protection of SGLT2 inhibitors in chronic kidney disease. Front Immunol 2021;12(2387):1–9.
62. Khazim K, Giustarini D, Rossi R, et al. Glutathione redox potential is low and glutathionylated and cysteinylated hemoglobin levels are elevated in maintenance hemodialysis patients. Transl Res 2013;162(1):16–25.
63. Kerns JC, Gutierrez JL. Thiamin. Adv Nutr 2017;8(2):395–7.
64. Marrs C, Lonsdale D. Hiding in plain sight: modern thiamine deficiency. Cells 2021;10(10):2595.
65. Thornalley P, Babaei-Jadidi R, Al Ali H, et al. High prevalence of low plasma thiamine concentration in diabetes linked to a marker of vascular disease. Diabetologia 2007;50(10):2164–70.
66. Mazzeo A, Barutta F, Bellucci L, et al. Reduced thiamine availability and hyperglycemia impair thiamine transport in renal glomerular cells through modulation of thiamine transporter 2. Biomedicines 2021;9(4).
67. Frank LL. Thiamin in clinical practice. J Parenter Enteral Nutr 2015;39(5):503–20.
68. Zhang F, Masania J, Anwar A, et al. The uremic toxin oxythiamine causes functional thiamine deficiency in end-stage renal disease by inhibiting transketolase activity. Kidney Int 2016;90(2):396–403.
69. Sambon M, Pavlova O, Alhama-Riba J, et al. Product inhibition of mammalian thiamine pyrophosphokinase is an important mechanism for maintaining thiamine

diphosphate homeostasis. Biochim Biophys Acta (Bba) - Gen Subjects 2022; 1866(3):130071.

70. Chazot C, Steiber AL, Kopple JD. Chapter 26 - Vitamin metabolism and requirements in chronic kidney disease and kidney failure. In: Kopple JD, Massry SG, Kalantar-Zadeh K, et al, editors. Nutritional management of renal disease. 4th edition. Academic Press; 2022. p. 413–65.

71. Long M, Zhu X, Wei X, et al. Magnesium in renal fibrosis. Int Urol Nephrol 2022; 54:1881–9.

72. Apetrii M, Covic A, Massy ZA. Chapter 22 - Magnesium and kidney disease. In: Kopple JD, Massry SG, Kalantar-Zadeh K, et al, editors. Nutritional management of renal disease. 4th edition. Academic Press; 2022. p. 345–51.

73. Galvan DL, Green NH, Danesh FR. The hallmarks of mitochondrial dysfunction in chronic kidney disease. Kidney Int 2017;92(5):1051–7.

74. Mafra D, Borges NA, Lindholm B, et al. Food as medicine: targeting the uraemic phenotype in chronic kidney disease. Nat Rev Nephrol 2021;17(3):153–71.

75. Ostrakhovitch EA, Tabibzadeh S. Chapter two - homocysteine in chronic kidney disease. In: Makowski GS, editor. Advances in clinical chemistryVol 72. Elsevier; 2015. p. 77–106.

76. Yu Y, Xiao L, Ren Z, et al. Glucose-induced decrease of cystathionine β-synthase mediates renal injuries. The FASEB J 2021;35(5):e21576.

77. Guerreiro Í, Ferreira-Pêgo C, Carregosa D, et al. Polyphenols and their metabolites in renal diseases: an overview. Foods 2022;11(7):1060.

78. Jones G, Strugnell SA and DeLuca HF, Current Understanding of the Molecular Actions of Vitamin D 1998, Physiological Reviews, 78, 1193–1231.

79. Antoniucci DM, Yamashita T, Portale AA. Dietary phosphorus regulates serum fibroblast growth factor-23 concentrations in healthy men. J Clin Endocrinol Metab 2006;91(8):3144–9.

80. Bellorin-Font E, Voinescu A, Martin KJ. Chapter 23 - Calcium, phosphate, PTH, vitamin D, and FGF-23 in CKD-mineral and bone disorder. In: Kopple JD, Massry SG, Kalantar-Zadeh K, et al, editors. Nutritional management of renal disease. 4th edition. Academic Press; 2022. p. 353–81.

81. Ettinger S. Essentials III - Nutrients for Bone Structure and Calcification. In: Ettinger S, editor. Nutritional pathophysiology of obesity and its comorbidities. Academic Press; 2017. p. 271–84.

82. Musgrove J, Wolf M. Regulation and Effects of FGF23 in Chronic Kidney Disease. Annu Rev Physiol 2020;82(1):365–90.

83. Fan Y, Liu W, Bi R, et al. Interrelated role of Klotho and calcium-sensing receptor in parathyroid hormone synthesis and parathyroid hyperplasia. Proc Natl Acad Sci 2018;115(16):E3749–58.

84. Grabner A, Amaral Ansel P, Schramm K, et al. Activation of Cardiac fibroblast growth factor receptor 4 causes left ventricular hypertrophy. Cell Metab 2015; 22(6):1020–32.

85. Bansal A, Chonchol M. Chapter 24 - Phosphorus metabolism and fibroblast growth factor 23 in chronic kidney disease. In: Kopple JD, Massry SG, Kalantar-Zadeh K, et al, editors. Nutritional management of renal disease. 4th edition. Academic Press; 2022. p. 383–96.

86. Tuominen M, Karp HJ, Itkonen ST. Phosphorus-containing food additives in the food supply—an audit of products on supermarket shelves. J Ren Nutr 2022; 32(1):30–8.

87. Borgi L. Inclusion of phosphorus in the nutrition facts label. Clin J Am Soc Nephrol 2019;14(1):139–40.

88. Carrero JJ, González-Ortiz A, Avesani CM, et al. Plant-based diets to manage the risks and complications of chronic kidney disease. Nat Rev Nephrol 2020;16(9): 525–42.

89. Board FaN. Dietary reference intakes: calcium, phosphorus, magnesium, vitamin D and fluoride. Washington (DC): National Academy Press; 1997.

90. Wei K-Y, Gritter M, Vogt L, et al. Dietary potassium and the kidney: lifesaving physiology. Clin Kidney J 2020;13(6):952–68.

91. Uhlig K, Berns JS, Kestenbaum B, et al. KDOQI US Commentary on the 2009 KDIGO Clinical Practice Guideline for the Diagnosis, Evaluation, and Treatment of CKD–Mineral and Bone Disorder (CKD-MBD). Am J Kidney Dis 2010;55(5): 773–99.

92. Ettinger S. Chapter 9 - osteoporosis and fracture risk. In: Ettinger S, editor. Nutritional pathophysiology of obesity and its comorbidities. Academic Press; 2017. p. 209–34.

93. Massy ZA, Drüeke TB. Magnesium and cardiovascular complications of chronic kidney disease. Nat Rev Nephrol 2015;11(7):432–42.

94. ter Braake AD, Tinnemans PT, Shanahan CM, et al. Magnesium prevents vascular calcification in vitro by inhibition of hydroxyapatite crystal formation. Scientific Rep 2018;8(1):2069.

95. Brandenburg VM, Kramann R, Specht P, et al. Calciphylaxis in CKD and beyond. Nephrol Dial Transplant 2012;27(4):1314–8.

96. Popa D-S, Bigman G, Rusu ME. The Role of Vitamin K in humans: implication in aging and age-associated diseases. Antioxidants 2021;10(4):566.

97. Danziger J. Vitamin K-dependent proteins, warfarin, and vascular calcification. Clin J Am Soc Nephrol 2008;3(5):1504–10.

98. Fusaro M, Cianciolo G, Evenepoel P, et al. Vitamin K in CKD Bone Disorders. Calcified Tissue Int 2021;108(4):476–85.

99. Schiefsky M. Hippocrates on ancient medicine - part 14: translated with introduction and commentary, 17. Brill; 2018 Jul.

Nutrition in Critically Ill Patients

Chelsea Jensen, MS, PA-C, RDN

KEYWORDS

• Nutrition • Critical illness • Critical care • Intensive care • Enteral nutrition

KEY POINTS

- Critical illness causes several metabolic changes. Providing early and adequate nutrition support may curtail some changes and lead to improved outcomes.
- Most patients will benefit from enteral nutrition. Parenteral nutrition should be reserved for specific cases only.
- Most patients will require 25 to 30 kcal/kg and 1.2 to 2 g/kg protein, but specific disease states may have other requirements.

INTRODUCTION

Critical illness is a large umbrella term that may encompass various forms of illness, from polytrauma, to renal failure, to sepsis, and so forth. However, regardless of the cause of critical illness, metabolic changes arise due to the stress inflicted on the body during these times. These changes can affect the healing and recovery processes during critical illness, which may lead to worse outcomes. Luckily, many of these changes may be curtailed by providing early and adequate nutrition, which results in both improved recovery time and functionality.[1] This article examines why nutrition is important in critical illness, how to determine who requires nutrition support, and how to provide nutrition support. In addition, barriers to nutrition support and how to overcome them as well as specific nutritional needs for several disease states are reviewed.

BACKGROUND: METABOLIC CHANGES DURING CRITICAL ILLNESS

The sequence of changes that occur during stress or critical illness has been described as the ebb, catabolic flow, and anabolic flow phases (**Fig. 1**). During the ebb phase, circulatory changes occur that require resuscitation, such as fluid, blood, or blood products. This usually occurs in the first 24 hours after injury. The catabolic flow phase occurs during the next 3 to 10 days after injury and is characterized by high levels of catabolism driven by cytokine mediators. The last phase,

Department of Neurosurgery, Neuroscience ICU, Northwell Health South Shore University Hospital, 301 East Main Street, Bay Shore, NY 11706, USA
E-mail address: cjjensen180@gmail.com

Physician Assist Clin 7 (2022) 701–712
https://doi.org/10.1016/j.cpha.2022.05.006
physicianassistant.theclinics.com

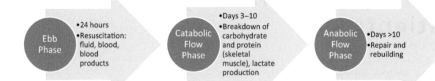

Fig. 1. Stages of critical illness. (Latifi R. Nutritional therapy in critically ill and injured patients. Surg Clin North Am. 2011;91(3):579-593; and Preiser JC, Ichai C, Orban JC, Groeneveld ABJ. Metabolic response to the stress of critical illness. Br J Anaesth. 2014;113(6):945-954.)

the anabolic flow phase, shows a shift in metabolism toward reparative processes and rebuilding.[2]

During the ebb and catabolic phases, uncontrolled catabolism is seen by carbohydrate breakdown, which occurs in addition to resistance to anabolic factors, such as insulin. This is a mechanism to provide glucose to vital organs rather than skeletal muscle and fat tissues. Lactate production is also increased to provide anaerobic metabolism of glucose. Last, protein breakdown is increased in skeletal muscle to provide energy to vital tissues. These processes combined may lead to a large increase in resting energy expenditure, hyperglycemia, and negative nitrogen balance.[3] Therefore, adequate nutrition is vital to help mediate these processes and aid in recovery from critical illness.

ASSESSING FOR NUTRITION RISK
Screening Tools

There are many ways to determine a patient's nutritional risk, but few are specifically provided for the critically ill patient. There are 2 scores that are most often used in critical illness, the Nutrition Risk Score (NRS) and the Nutrition Risk in Critically Ill (NUTRIC) score.

The NRS is a validated tool for determining nutritional risk in patients ages 18 to 90. The score considers body mass index (BMI), recent weight loss, reduced dietary intake, critical illness status, and severity of disease.[4] Although this score adjusts for critical illness, it was not specifically made for those critically ill. In contrast, the NUTRIC score was designed specifically for the critically ill. This tool uses the patient's age, APACHE II (Acute Physiology and Chronic Health Evaluation) score, SOFA (Sepsis-related Organ Failure Assessment) score, number of comorbidities, days from intensive care unit (ICU) admission, and interleukin-6, if available. Patients are then classified as "high" nutrition risk versus "low" nutrition risk.[5] Per the American Society for Parenteral and Enteral Nutrition (ASPEN) recommendations, the NUTRIC score is the best tool to determine an individual patient's nutritional risk and need for aggressive nutritional intervention.[1]

Serum Markers

Historically, serum markers, such as albumin, prealbumin, transferrin, and the like, have been used as a marker for nutritional status. However, these markers are not validated for use in critical illness. These markers are acute phase reactants that are altered in critical illness and do not represent nutritional status in ICU settings; therefore, they should not be used.[1,6]

ESTIMATING NUTRITION NEEDS
Calories

There are many ways to measure or estimate a patient's caloric needs. The most accurate method is to perform indirect calorimetry (IC).[1] Unfortunately, most facilities do not have access to or staffing for performing IC on every critically ill patient.

There are several equations that have been developed to estimate a patient's daily caloric needs, including weight-based equations, Harris-Benedict, Mifflin, Penn State, and Ireton-Jones, to name a few. However, several studies have shown that when measured against IC in a critically ill patient, no one equation is superior to the others.[1,7,8] Therefore, ASPEN recommends using weight-based equations owing to their simplicity. Most patients will require 25 to 30 kcal/kg actual body weight (ABW), although there is new evidence to show that there is no significant difference in outcomes between higher and lower caloric intake (12–25 kcal/kg).[9] Adjustments for obesity are detailed in later discussions.

Protein

Protein is the most important nutrient to help maintain lean body mass (LBM), immune function, and wound healing,[1] and negative nitrogen balance has been associated with higher mortality and poor functional outcomes.[10] For most patients, providing 1.2 to 2 g/kg of ABW is sufficient to maintain LBM and prevent skeletal muscle mass loss. Protein intake should be optimized, even when patients are not meeting their calorie needs, and protein supplementation may be required.[1,9]

Nitrogen balance studies have been used in research settings to monitor protein intake and losses. However, their use and practicality in ICU settings are limited.[1]

WHEN TO INITIATE NUTRITION SUPPORT

Nutrition support should be started as soon as possible, ideally within the first 24 to 48 hours in those who cannot maintain adequate oral intake. Enteral nutrition (EN) is preferred over parenteral nutrition (PN) owing to its advantageous effects, including maintaining gut integrity, modulating the stress and immune responses, and decreasing disease severity.[1] A review by Marik and Zaloga[11] indicated that patients who were provided early EN (<24 hours) had lower rates of infections (RR, 0.45; $P = .00006$) and reduced hospital length of stay (LOS) (−2.2 days; $P = .0012$). Another review, by Doig and colleagues,[12] also demonstrated that early EN (<24 hours) had a significant reduction in pneumonia (OR, 0.31; $P = .001$) and mortality (OR, 0.34; $P = .02$). An additional report by Mizuma and colleagues[13] shows that early EN, within 48 hours, reduces the risk of pneumonia (28.1% in late EN vs 8.5% in early EN; $P<.001$). Last, meeting protein goals by day 4 has been shown to have lower surgical complications and reduce the number of operations needed.[14]

FEEDING METHODS
Enteral Nutrition

Gastrointestinal versus small bowel feeding
There has been debate about ideal placement of EN access, and each has its own merits and flaws. Gastric enteral feeding is easier to place and decreases time to initiation of nutrition. However, delivery to the small intestine (nasoduodenal or nasojejunal) has improved nutrient delivery and reduced risk of pneumonia.[1] Several reviews have compared prepyloric versus postpyloric feedings and their complications and outcomes with conflicting results. Sajid and colleagues[15] found that postpyloric feeding had lower gastric residual volumes and higher calorie delivery, whereas

gastric feedings had a higher risk for aspiration. Another review article found that there was no difference in energy delivery or incidence of pneumonia between gastric and postpyloric feeding.[16] ASPEN recommends postpyloric feedings if a patient is at high risk for aspiration or has an intolerance to gastric feedings, but otherwise, gastric feedings are sufficient to provide early initiation of EN.[1]

Feeding rates and administration

Any type of feeding, whether trophic feeds or full feeds providing greater than 80% of estimated nutritional needs, is superior to no nutritional supplementation. Trophic feeding generally provides less than 500 kcal/d or less than 15% to 25% of the patient's estimated needs, and there is evidence to show that trophic feeds may prevent gut atrophy and maintain gut integrity in patients with low nutritional risk. In contrast, those at high nutrition risk or severe malnutrition should have feedings advanced to greater than 80% of needs over 24 to 48 hours while monitoring for refeeding syndrome.[1] However, other sources have found that there is no significant difference between trophic and full feeding. Phan and colleagues[17] found that there was no significant difference in mortality, length of mechanical ventilation, or hospital LOS between trophic and full feeding, and Wang and colleagues[18] found that there was no difference in mortality.

Whether providing trophic or full feeding, feeding regimen may vary between hourly feeding rates versus volume feeding protocols. Although hourly feeding has been used most traditionally, there is now emerging evidence that volume-based protocols may be superior. Two separate randomized control trials have demonstrated that volume-based feeding provides a higher percentage of goal calories compared with hourly-based feeding and that no significant differences in vomiting, regurgitation, feeding intolerance, or diarrhea occurred.[19,20] Volume-based feedings may provide more adequate nutrition with no difference in subsequent complications.

Parenteral Nutrition

The use of PN, its initiation, its duration of use, and other considerations have been the topic of debate for years. Although there are benefits to using PN, there are also many side effects. Per ASPEN guidelines, if a patient is at low nutritional risk, PN should be held until days 7 to 10 and can then be initiated if the patient is unable to maintain oral intake and/or tolerate EN. If the patient is at high nutritional risk and is unable to tolerate EN, PN should be started immediately. However, PN should be started slowly and advanced to provide goal calories over 3 to 4 days with some sources recommending less than 20 kcal/kg with adequate protein to be provided over the first week.[1] While providing PN, the medical team should be monitoring for signs of refeeding syndrome, hyperglycemia, and infection. The patient should be transitioned to EN as soon as possible. PN may also be provided as an adjunct to EN if the patient is unable to meet his/her nutritional needs with EN alone.

Oral Nutrition

Most critically ill patients require EN or PN at some point during their medical course, but as patients improve, most will transition to oral nutrition. Providing oral nutrition has many barriers, including swallowing function and diet consistency, patient food preferences, and poor appetite to name a few. A study by Rougier and colleagues[21] found that orally fed patients on average consumed only 9.7 kcal/kg/d and 0.35 g/kg/d protein, which is far below most recommendations. Providing adequate nutrition in these patients is just as critical as in those receiving EN or PN.

Calorie counts have been used to track oral intakes to determine calorie and protein consumed. This may be beneficial to determine if a patient needs further nutrition intervention, such as supplemental oral or EN. The use of oral nutrition supplements is also common in the intensive care setting and can be extremely advantageous. However, their benefits are only helpful if the patient is willing to consume the supplement. In some cases, supplemental EN may be preferred to decrease the patient's burden on oral intake, while allowing patients to receive adequate nutrition therapy to aid in their recovery.

COMPLICATIONS
Diarrhea

Diarrhea is a complication of EN administration and can contribute to electrolyte imbalance, skin breakdown, and wound contamination.[1] There are many factors associated with diarrhea in the critically ill patient, including type and amount of fiber in the enteral formula, osmolality of the enteral formula, patient medications, including antibiotics, proton-pump inhibitors, prokinetics, nonsteroidal anti-inflammatories, laxatives, and so forth, as well as infection. In a study by Sripongpun and colleagues,[22] the investigators found that the most common cause of diarrhea was medications (61.3% of cases), whereas EN was the cause in only 6.5% of cases. Unfortunately, EN is most often the scapegoat and is stopped, which then affects the patient's nutritional status. Rather than holding EN, feeds should continue while the cause of diarrhea is determined and addressed.

Both fiber and probiotics have been investigated in their relation to diarrhea. Zhao and colleagues[23] found that in patients with gastric cancer, a fiber-enriched formula had decreased incidence of diarrhea compared with no fiber supplementation ($P = .007$), and a diet enriched with both fiber and a probiotic had even lower incidences of diarrhea ($P = .003$). Rushdi and colleagues[24] also found fewer liquid stools when soluble fiber was added ($P<.01$). ASPEN recommends that in stable critically ill patients, a fermentable soluble fiber additive may be beneficial, but it should be avoided in those at high risk for bowel ischemia or severe dysmotility.[1]

Aspiration

Aspiration is one of the most feared complications of EN. Risks of aspiration include nasoenteric tubes, poor oral care, mechanical ventilation, age greater than 70 years old, supine position, neurologic deficits, gastroesophageal reflux, and transport in and out of the ICU. However, it is much more common for aspiration to be from oral secretions than from EN.[1] In those at high risk of aspiration, postpyloric feeding is recommended. If the patient remains with prepyloric feeding, continuous infusion is recommended. Promotility agents, such as metoclopramide and erythromycin, may also be used with caution taken in regard to their side effects. Aspiration can be reduced by keeping the head of bed between 30° and 45° and ensuring good oral hygiene.[1]

Refeeding Syndrome

Refeeding syndrome is common in the critically ill population, especially in those at high nutritional risk. Refeeding syndrome occurs in patients with baseline malnutrition during the shift from catabolism to anabolism after feeding is initiated. During the fasting/catabolic state, intracellular electrolytes are depleted, but extracellular concentrations are maintained. When feeding is initiated and anabolism begins, electrolytes are then shifted intracellularly and cause extracellular depletion. This can lead to cardiac, respiratory, hematologic, gastrointestinal, neurologic, and musculoskeletal complications.[25]

There have been several definitions of refeeding syndrome, ranging from hypophosphatemia alone to fluid abnormalities and organ dysfunction. ASPEN provided their definition as the extent of decrease in serum electrolytes (phosphate, magnesium, potassium): mild: 10% to 20% decrease; moderate: 20% to 30% decrease; and severe: greater than 30% decrease and/or organ dysfunction. Refeeding syndrome may occur within hours or up to 5 days after increasing nutrition.[26] Several studies have shown that refeeding syndrome occurs in 17% to 37% of critically ill patients.[27,28] Those at high nutrition risk were more likely to develop refeeding syndrome, and it was associated with longer ICU LOS, and higher 30-day and 6-month mortality.[27]

Per ASPEN recommendations, those at risk for refeeding syndrome should have their nutrition support initiated at a maximum of 40% to 50% of energy goals, and monitoring of serum electrolytes should take place every 12 hours for the first 3 days in the high-risk patient with repletion as appropriate. Thiamine and multivitamin supplementation should also be provided.[26]

NUTRITION IN SPECIFIC DISEASE STATES
Renal Failure

Kidney injury is a common complication of critical illness, with more than 50% of ICU patients developing it.[29] Although kidney injury is common, most patients will not require specialty nutrition formulas or adjustments to estimated needs. Most sources recommend using 25 to 30 kcal/kg dry weight for calorie needs and 1.2 to 2 g/kg dry weight for protein needs for patients not requiring renal replacement therapy (RRT).[1,30] Standard EN formulas should also be sufficient, but if a patient does develop significant electrolyte abnormalities, a renal-specific formula may be used.[30]

Patients who are undergoing RRT have other nutritional considerations. RRT extracts significant amounts of protein during filtration, and thus patients require higher protein administration. Most sources suggest a range of 1.5 to 2.5 g/kg to maintain protein stores.[1,31] Patients who require continuous RRT have an increased uptake of glucose and citrate up to 500 kcal/d.[32] This may lead to overfeeding in critically ill patients, so care should be taken when determining a patient's nutritional needs (**Table 1**).

Hepatic Failure

Liver failure presents a few barriers to providing adequate nutrition. Liver failure often leads to edema and ascites, which may make energy and protein calculations inaccurate. If available, IC is preferred to determine energy needs, but if unavailable, dry weight or usual weight should be used for calculations.[1] General nutrition calculations should be used, with goal energy needs as 25 to 30 kcal/kg.[1,33] Some sources do recommend higher calorie needs with the range of 35 to 40 kcal/kg,[33] but this may lead to overfeeding.

Liver failure is often complicated by encephalopathy owing to increased ammonia levels, which is a byproduct of protein breakdown. In the past, some practitioners have advocated for protein restriction to reduce risk of encephalopathy developing, but new evidence suggests that protein restrictions do not reduce encephalopathy and may lead to skeletal muscle mass loss. Current studies recommend 1.2 to 1.5 g/kg to meet protein needs.[1,33] Specialty formulas exist that provide branched chain amino acids (BCAAs) to avoid protein breakdown and ammonia production. There is some evidence that using a BCAA-rich formula may improve hepatic encephalopathy,[34] but current recommendations suggest using generalized, concentrated (1.5 kcal/mL) formulas. If encephalopathy does develop, then a BCAA-rich formula may be used (**Table 1**).[1,33]

Pancreatitis

Pancreatitis complicates nutrition support possibly more than any other disease state because the pancreas provides many enzymes necessary for nutrition breakdown and absorption. Because of this, many providers lean toward restricting nutrition support or providing PN first. However, Wu and colleagues[35] found that providing EN over PN reduces mortality (RR, 0.43; P = .006), reduces hospital LOS (-2.93 days; P = .0001), and lowers the risk of infection and other complications (RR, 0.53; P = .0001). Therefore, providing oral and/or EN is preferred over PN.

For mild pancreatitis, an oral diet should be provided. If oral intake is insufficient after 7 days, then EN may be started. For moderate to severe pancreatitis, EN should be initiated as trophic feedings and advanced to goal over 24 to 48 hours.[1] Prepyloric and postpyloric feeding access has shown no difference in pancreatitis patients regarding mortality, multiorgan failure, infection, or need for surgical intervention.[1,36] Therefore, EN access should be established as soon as possible. If a patient has poor tolerance to EN, feeding access can be advanced more distally in the gastrointestinal tract; continuous infusion can be used, or a formula of small peptide or medium-chain triglyceride formula may be helpful.[1]

PN should be avoided if the patient is able to tolerate EN.[1] However, if a patient is unable to tolerate EN or is not meeting nutritional needs with EN alone, PN may be necessary. PN should only be provided in severe pancreatitis and after 24 to 48 hours of full liquid resuscitation. Evidence has shown that providing PN versus no nutritional support has reduced complications, hospital LOS, and overall mortality (**Table 1**).[1]

Polytrauma

Polytrauma can complicate providing adequate nutrition in several ways. Hormone changes after trauma promote skeletal muscle loss early with up to 16% of total body protein being depleted within the first 21 days.[1] Resting energy expenditure peaks on days 4 to 5 after trauma but may remain elevated for up to 9 to 12 days. Because of this, providing early nutrition with a focus on protein is vital to maintaining the patient's LBM. As with other disease states, early EN is recommended within 24 to 48 hours if hemodynamically stable. Calorie goals should be between 20 and 35 kcal/kg, and protein recommendations remain at 1.2 to 2 g/kg.[1]

Many providers may be hesitant to use EN owing to the patient's overall trauma. However, there are many injuries when EN is still appropriate, including open abdomen, mild ileus, new ostomy, prone positioning, and use of neuromuscular blockade. Conditions that would not be appropriate for EN include intestinal discontinuity, obstruction, ischemic bowel, high output fistula, or high use of vasopressors.[37] In these cases, PN would be appropriate until the patient is able to tolerate EN (**Table 1**).

Traumatic Brain Injury

Traumatic brain injury (TBI) is a subset of trauma. However, because of the traumatic effects on the brain, the metabolic changes and requirements are somewhat different from generalized trauma. TBI can alter the patient's basal metabolic rate, with some increases up to 200%, after injury; therefore, providing early nutrition, adequate calories, and protein is essential. Patients with TBI should have EN initiated within 24 to 48 hours, and protein recommendations are 1.5 to 2.5 g/kg.[1] Hartl and colleagues[38] found that patients who did not receive nutrition after 5 and 7 days had a two- and four-fold increase in mortality, respectively. They also found that the amount of nutrition provided was directly related to mortality, with every 10 kcal/kg decrease in energy intake increasing risk of mortality by 30% to 40%. Chapple and colleagues[39] also found that patients with greater energy and protein deficits had longer ICU and hospital LOS (P<.001). A study performed by Yang and colleagues[40] found that patients who received adequate nutrition support had decreased rates of general infection (RR, 0.54; P<.0001), lung infections (RR, 0.60; P = .0006), ICU LOS (−5.65 days; P<.00001), and improved Glasgow Coma Scales (2.77; P<.00001) (**Table 1**).

Burns

Burns cause several metabolic changes similar to general trauma, but the magnitude and duration of injury are far worse, and nutrition support is vital to help prevent infection, loss of LBM, and overall mortality.[41] Because of the hypermetabolic state of burns, it is very difficult to accurately assess calorie needs; therefore, IC is recommended for all burn patients if available.[1] If IC is unavailable, 25 kcal/kg plus 40 kcal per percent body area burned should be provided.[41] Protein goals should range between 1.5 and 2 g/kg.[1]

Early nutrition support should be initiated in all burn patients, ideally within 4 to 6 hours of injury. EN should be used in those whose gastrointestinal tracts are functional, and PN should be used for those in which EN is not tolerated or as an adjunct to EN.[1] Early EN (<24 hours) has been shown to reduce morality (OR, 0.36; P = .003), gastrointestinal hemorrhage (OR, 0.21; P = .0005), sepsis (OR, 0.23; P<.0001), pneumonia (OR, 0.41; P = .01), renal failure (OR, 0.27; P = .002), and hospital LOS (−15.31 days; P<.0001) in major burn patients (**Table 1**).[42]

Sepsis

Patients with sepsis often have other underlying organ dysfunction, but sepsis itself causes metabolic derangements and need for nutritional support. EN is recommended over PN and can be initiated within 24 to 48 hours after resuscitation is completed and the patient is hemodynamically stable.[1] It is recommended to start trophic feeds during the initial phase of sepsis with increasing toward goal calories over the first week, with some evidence showing that providing even 25% to 66% of calories is sufficient.[1,43] Protein recommendations include 1.2 to 2 g/kg.[1]

PN is not recommended in early severe or septic shock, regardless of nutrition risk. If PN is required, late initiation (>8 days after ICU admission) is recommended. If PN is initiated early (within 48 hours), there is a higher risk of infection, longer ICU and hospital LOS, and longer duration of organ dysfunction (**Table 1**).[44]

Postoperative

Postoperative patients are an interesting subset of critically ill patients. Even though some postoperative patients underwent elective surgery, the metabolic changes that occur are similar to other critical illnesses. Therefore, EN is again recommended over PN in most cases, including prolonged ileus, intestinal anastomosis, open abdomen, and pressor requirements.[1] EN should be initiated within 24 hours after surgery. In some cases where EN is not suitable, PN should be initiated only if it will be required for greater than 7 days; if not, nutrition should be held and EN initiated within 5 to 7 days.[1]

If a patient can tolerate oral nutrition, clear liquids are not required as the first meal. Studies have shown that early initiation of solid food improves motility and bowel function and is recommended as tolerated (**Table 1**).[1]

Table 1
Summary of disease states and nutrition recommendations

Disease State	Energy Needs	Protein Needs	Other Recommendations
Renal failure	25–30 kcal/kg dry weight	No RRT: 1.2–2 g/kg RRT: 1.5–2.5 g/kg	Monitor for overfeeding if on continuous RRT
Hepatic failure	25–30 kcal/kg dry weight	1.2–1.5 g/kg	May use BCAA-rich formula if develop encephalopathy
Pancreatitis	25–30 kcal/kg	1.2–2 g/kg	Moderately severe: Start trophic, advance >24–48 h Prepyloric vs postpyloric feeding no difference
Polytrauma	20–35 kcal/kg	1.2–2 g/kg	
TBI	25–30 kcal/kg	1.5–2.5 g/kg	
Burns	25 kcal/kg + 40 kcal per % surface body area burned	1.5–2 g/kg	
Sepsis	25–30 kcal/kg	1.2–2 g/kg	Start trophic, increase to goal kcals over 1 wk PN should not be used in early severe or septic shock
Postoperative	25–30 kcal/kg	1.2–2 g/kg	PN not used unless required >7 d
Obesity	BMI 35–50: 11–14 kcal/kg ABW BMI >50: 22–25 kcal/kg IBW	BMI 30–40: 2 g/kg IBW BMI >40: 2.5 g/kg IBW	Some gradual weight loss during admission may be beneficial

Obesity

Although obesity is not a critical illness itself, obesity complicates many aspects of the critically ill patient's care and treatment. Because a patient has obesity, a practitioner may believe that they cannot be malnourished or require early nutrition; however, this is a false notion. Patients with obesity have a high rate of malnutrition and require early nutrition (within 24–48 hours). Indications of high-risk patients include those with central adiposity, metabolic syndrome, sarcopenia, BMI greater than 40, systemic inflammatory response syndrome, and other comorbidities.[1]

Hypocaloric, high-protein feedings are recommended to preserve LBM, mobilize adipose stores, and reduce complications of overfeeding.[1] Energy and protein needs are difficult to calculate in these patients, but weight-based equations are still recommended with some adjustments. For a patient with BMI of 35 to 50, a goal of 11 to 14 kcal/kg ABW is recommended; for BMI greater than 50, a goal of 22 to 25 kcal/kg ideal body weight (IBW) is recommended. Protein goals are also adjusted: BMI of 30 to 40, protein recommendations include 2 g/kg IBW; BMI greater than 40, 2.5 g/kg IBW is recommended.[1] Some weight loss during admission may be beneficial, with improvements in insulin sensitivity, nursing care, and reduced comorbidities; therefore, some component of weight loss may be acceptable during admission (**Table 1**).

SUMMARY

Critical illness causes several metabolic changes, many of which affect nutritional status. Numerous studies demonstrate that providing adequate nutrition during critical illness improves patient outcomes and overall recovery. Most patients will benefit from EN over PN. Although there may be barriers to providing nutrition, such as diarrhea or risk of aspiration, continued nutrition support is recommended. Specific disease states have varying nutrition recommendations, but most important is providing early (within 24–48 hours) and adequate (>80% energy and protein needs) nutrition to aid in healing.

CLINICS CARE POINTS

- Early nutrition support (within 24–48 hours) is recommended.
- Enteral nutrition is preferred over parenteral nutrition in most critically ill patients.
- Most patients require 25 to 30 kcal/kg and 1.2 to 2 g/kg protein, although specific disease states may vary slightly in recommendations.

DISCLOSURE

The author has nothing to disclose.

REFERENCES

1. McClave SA, Taylor BE, Martindale RG, et al. Guidelines for the provision and assessment of nutrition support therapy in the adult critically ill patients. J Parenter Enteral Nutr 2016;40(2):159–211.
2. Latifi R. Nutritional therapy in critically ill and injured patients. Surg Clin North Am 2011;91(3):579–93.
3. Preiser JC, Ichai C, Orban JC, et al. Metabolic response to the stress of critical illness. Br J Anaesth 2014;113(6):945–54.
4. Kondrup J, Rasmussen HH, Hamberg O, et al. Nutritional risk screening (NRS 2002): a new method based on an analysis of controlled clinical trials. Clin Nutr 2003;22(3):321–36.
5. Rahman A, Hasan RM, Agarwala R, et al. Identifying critically-ill patients who will benefit most from nutritional therapy: Further validation of the "modified NUTRIC" nutritional risk assessment tool. Clin Nutr 2016;35(1):158–62.
6. Davis CJ, Sowa D, Keim KS, et al. The use of prealbumin and c-reactive protein for monitoring nutrition support in adult patients receiving enteral nutrition in an urban medical center. J Parenter Enteral Nutr 2011;36(2):197–204.
7. Frankenfield DC, Coleman A, Alam S, et al. Analysis of estimation methods for resting metabolic rate in critically ill adults. J Parenter Enteral Nutr 2009;33(1):27–36.
8. Faisy C, Guerot E, Diehl JL, et al. Assessment of resting energy expenditure in mechanically ventilated patients. Am J Clin Nutr 2003;78(2):241–9.
9. Compher C, Bingham A, McCall M, et al. Guidelines for the provision of nutrition support therapy in the adult critically ill patient: The American Society for Parenteral and Enteral Nutrition. JPEN J Parenter Enteral Nutr 2022;46(1):12–41.
10. Kim TJ, Park SH, Jeong HB, et al. Optimizing nitrogen balance is associated with better outcomes in neurocritically ill patients. Nutrients 2020;12:3137.
11. Marik PE, Zaloga GP. Early enteral nutrition in acutely ill patients: a systematic review. Crit Care Med 2001;29(12):2264–70.
12. Doig GS, Heighes PT, Simpson F, et al. Early enteral nutrition, provided within 24 h of injury or intensive care unit admission, significantly reduces mortality in

critically ill patients; a meta-analysis of randomised control trials. Intensive Care Med 2009;35(12):2018–27.

13. Mizuma A, Netsu S, Sakamoto M, et al. Effect of early enteral nutrition on critical care outcomes in patients with acute ischemic stroke. J Int Med Res 2021; 49(11):1–12.

14. Hartwell J, Cotton A, Wenos C, et al. Early achievement of enteral nutrition protein goals by intensive care unit day 4 is associated with fewer complications in critically injured adults. Ann Surg 2021;274(6):e988–94.

15. Sajid MS, Harper A, Hussain Q, et al. An integrated systematic review and meta-analysis of published and randomized controlled trials evaluating nasogastric against postpyloris (nasoduodenal and nasojejunal) feeding in critically ill patients admitted in intensive care unit. Eur J Clin Nutr 2014;68:424–32.

16. Davies AR, Morrison SS, Bailey MJ, et al. A multicenter, randomized controlled trial comparing early nasojejunal with nasogastric nutrition in critical illness. Crit Care Med 2012;40(8):2342–8.

17. Phan KA, Dux CM, Osland EJ, et al. Effect of hypocaloric normoprotein or trophic feeding versus target full feeding on patient outcomes in critically ill adults: a systematic review. Anaesth Intensive Care 2017;45(6):663–75.

18. Wang CY, Fu PK, Chao WC, et al. Full versus trophic feeds in critically ill adults with high and low nutritional risk scores: a randomized control trial. Nutrients 2020;12:3518.

19. Sachdev G, Backes K, Thomas BW, et al. Volume-based protocol improves delivery of enteral nutrition in critically ill trauma patients. J Parenter Enteral Nutr 2020;44(5):874–9.

20. McClave SA, Saad MA, Esterle M, et al. Volume-based feeding in the critically ill patient. J Parenter Enteral Nutr 2015;39(6):707–12.

21. Rougier L, Preiser JC, Fadeur M, et al. Nutrition during critical care: an audit on actual energy and protein intakes. J Parenter Enteral Nutr 2021;45(5):951–60.

22. Sripongpun P, Lertpipopmetha K, Chamroonkul N, et al. Diarrhea in tube-fed hospitalized patients: feeding formula is not the most common cause. J Gastroenterol Heptaol 2021;36(9):2441–7.

23. Zhao R, Want Y, Huang Y, et al. Effects of fiber and probiotics on diarrhea associated with enteral nutrition in gastric cancer patients: a prospective randomized control trial. Med 2017;96(43):e8418.

24. Rushdi TA, Pichard C, Khater YH. Control of diarrhea by fiber-enriched diet in ICU patients on enteral nutrition: a prospective randomized control trial. Clin Nutr 2004;23(6):1344–52.

25. Ponzo V, Pellegrini M, Cioffi I, et al. The refeeding syndrome: a neglected but potentially serious condition for inpatients. A narrative review. Intern Emerg Med 2021;16:49–60.

26. Da Silva JSV, Seres DS, Sabino K, et al. ASPEN consensus recommendations for refeeding syndrome. Nutr Clin Pract 2020;35(2):178–95.

27. Xiong R, Huang H, Wu Y, et al. Incidence and outcome of refeeding syndrome in neurocritically ill patients. Clin Nutr 2021;40(3):1071–6.

28. Olthof LE, Koekkoek WACK, van Setten C, et al. Impact of caloric intake in critically ill patients with, and without, refeeding syndrome: a retrospective study. Clin Nutr 2018;37(5):1609–17.

29. Ronco C, Bellomo R, Kellum JA. Acute kidney injury. Lancet 2019;394(10212): 1949–64.

30. Fiaccadori E, Regolisti G, Maggiore U. Specialized nutritional support interventions in critically ill patients on renal replacement therapy. Curr Opin Clin Nutr Metab Care 2013;16(2):217–24.

31. Scheinkestel CD, Kar L, Marshall K, et al. Prospective randomized trial to assess caloric and protein needs of critically ill, anuric, ventilated patients requiring continuous renal replacement therapy. Nutr 2003;19(11–12):909–16.

32. New AM, Nystrom EM, Frazee E, et al. Continuous renal replacement therapy: a potential source of calories in the critically ill. Am J Clin Nutr 2017;105(6):1559–63.

33. Kerwin AJ, Nussbaum MS. Adjuvant nutrition management of patients with liver failure, including transplant. Surg Clin North Am 2011;91(3):565–78.

34. Milan H. Branched-chain amino acids and ammonia metabolism in liver disease: therapeutic implications. Nutr 2013;29(10):1186–91.

35. Wu P, Li L, Sun W. Efficacy comparisons of enteral nutrition and parenteral nutrition in patients with severe acute pancreatitis: a meta-analysis from randomized controlled trials. Biosci Rep 2018;38(6):1–9.

36. Dutta AK, Goel A, Kirubakaran R, et al. Nasogastric versus nasojejunal tube feeding for severe acute pancreatitis. Cochrane Database Syst Rev 2020;3(3):CD010582.

37. Hartwell J, Peck K, Ley EJ, et al. Nutrition therapy in the critically injured adult patient: A Western Trauma Association critical decisions algorithm. J Trauma Acute Care Surg 2021;91(5):909–15.

38. Hartl R, Gerber LM, Ni Q, et al. Effect of early nutrition on deaths due to severe traumatic brain injury. J Neurosurg 2008;109(1):50–6.

39. Chapple LS, Chapman MJ, Lange K, et al. Nutrition support practices in critically ill head-injured patients: a global perspective. Crit Care 2015;20(6):1–12.

40. Yang L, Liao D, Hou X, et al. Systematic review and meta-analysis of the effect of nutritional support on the clinical outcome of patients with traumatic brain injury. Ann Palliat Med 2021;10(11):11960–9.

41. Williams FN, Branski LK, Jeschke MG, et al. What, how, and how much should burn patients be fed? Surg Clin North Am 2011;91(3):609–29.

42. Pu H, Doig G, Heighes PT, et al. Early enteral nutrition reduces mortality and improves other key outcomes in patients with major burn injury: a meta-analysis of randomized control trials. Crit Care Med 2018;46(12):2036–42.

43. Stapleton RD, Jones N, Heyland DK. Feeding critically ill patients: what is the optimal amount of energy? Crit Care Med 2007;35(9):S535–40.

44. Casaer MP, Mesotten D, Hermans G, et al. Early versus late parenteral nutrition in critically ill adults. N Engl J Med 2011;365:506–17.

Nutritional Care for the Older Adult

Melissa Bernstein, PhD, RDN, LD, DipACLM[a],*, Jay Bernstein, MD, MPH, MS[b]

KEYWORDS

- Sarcopenia • Sarcopenic obesity • Food desert • Food security
- Medical nutrition therapy (MNT)

KEY POINTS

- The goal for nutritional health in adults at every age should be to preserve physical and mental well-being and maintain a high quality of life.
- Consumption of a high-quality, nutritious diet is essential to optimize health and well-being at any age.
- Consuming a nutritious diet is influenced by health status and factors that may occur naturally with aging, or as a result of illness; this can interfere with an older adult's ability to meet their nutritional needs, especially when calorie needs are reduced.
- Routine screening for nutrition-related conditions such as malnutrition, frailty, sarcopenia, and sarcopenic obesity can lead to early intervention and prevention of worsening health outcomes.
- Many factors influence food intake in this population; therefore, individualized guidance is necessary to help older adults overcome medical, physical, economic, and social barriers to eating a healthy diet.

INTRODUCTION

Nutritional health is widely accepted as a key determinant of successful aging. Compared with younger adults, older adults are at greater risk of chronic diseases, such as cardiovascular disease, and cancer, as well as health conditions related to changes in bone and muscle mass, such as osteoporosis and sarcopenia. To reduce the burden of chronic disease and promote healthy aging, all adults must adopt healthy lifestyle practices and dietary habits. Adequate nutritional intake is critical for promoting well-being, maintenance of functional status, and preventing malnutrition and related comorbidities such as acute and chronic illness. Common

[a] Department of Nutrition, Rosalind Franklin University of Medicine and Science, 3333 Green Bay Road, North Chicago, IL 60064, USA; [b] Department of Emergency Medicine, Boonshoft School of Medicine, Wright State University, 2555 University Boulevard Suite 110, Fairborn, OH 45324, USA
* Corresponding author.
E-mail address: melissa.bernstein@rosalindfranklin.edu

Physician Assist Clin 7 (2022) 713–726
https://doi.org/10.1016/j.cpha.2022.06.003
physicianassistant.theclinics.com

complications in old age such as the increased burden of poor health, polypharmacy, reduced socialization, and limited functional ability can contribute to poor nutritional status. This review introduces some of the requirements, challenges, clinical considerations, and services needed to promote optimal nutritional intake for older adults.

DEMOGRAPHICS OF THE AGING POPULATION

Older adults are the largest growing group in the United States, representing 16% of the population.[1] Aging baby boomers enjoy a longer life span and will contribute to the near doubling of the 65 years and older population of Americans anticipated over the next 40 years, from 52 million in 2018 to 80.8 million by 2040.[2] The population aged 85 years and older is projected to more than double from 6.6 million in 2019 to 14.4 million in 2040 representing a 118% increase.[1] By 2060 almost a quarter of the US population will be aged 65 years or older.[3]

DIETARY GUIDANCE FOR OLDER ADULTS

Lifestyle behaviors including a healthy diet early in life have a dramatic and lasting impact on health in later years. The goal of nutrition recommendations in the aging population is the maintenance of a nutrient-dense diet to promote health and prevent nutrition-related complications that could contribute to declining health, functional dependency, and frailty. Each adult arrives at old age with different nutritional requirements built on lifelong dietary behaviors and other aspects of health status. Individualized patient care is essential from all members of the interprofessional health care team because the nutritional needs and challenges are as unique as the older adults themselves.

Healthy older adults are encouraged to follow the same dietary recommendations as those provided for the general adult population on the types of foods and beverages that comprise a healthy dietary pattern as described in the *Dietary Guidelines for Americans 2020 to 2025*.[4] However, from 2001 to 2018, the proportion of older adults with poor diet quality has increased from 51% to 61% and older adults with an ideal diet stayed consistently low at 0.4%.[5] Similar to other age groups, the actual average daily intake of total fruit, total vegetables, dairy foods, and seafood falls below the recommended intake ranges and exceeds limits for added sugar, saturated fat, and sodium in the United States.[4] Evidence suggests that plant-based diets that minimize processed foods can support a high quality of life as people age.[6] MyPlate (**Box 1**) recommendations for older adults are tailored to address the unique needs for individuals

---

Box 1
The US Department of Agriculture MyPlate for older adults emphasizes

- Enjoying a variety of nutrient-dense food choices such as protein-rich foods, plenty of vegetables, fruits, whole grains, healthy oils, and low-fat dairy choices
- Drinking water often to stay hydrated
- Choosing foods with little or no added sugar, saturated fat, and sodium
- Maintaining a healthy body weight
- Regular physical activity
- Food safety

https://www.myplate.gov/life-stages/older-adults.

older than 60 years, includes nutrition tips specific for this age group that addresses common barriers to a nutritious diet, and provides resources to help older adults.[7]

DISCUSSION
Nutrient Recommendations and Requirements

Energy
Older adults generally have lower calorie needs but similar or even increased nutrient needs compared with younger adults, therefore, the overall nutrient density of dietary patterns is particularly important to this age group. Eating nutritious food without over-consuming calories can be a challenge in the face of functional dependence, frailty, and illness. Older adults who do not reduce their caloric intake to balance a decrease in energy expenditure are at risk for overweight, obesity, and associated complications, metabolic consequences, and comorbidities.[8]

Energy intake and energy requirements commonly decline with advancing age. Lower caloric energy requirements result from decreased energy expenditure, losses in lean body mass, and reduced physical activity. Women aged 60 years and older require about 1600 to 2200 calories per day, and men aged 60 years and older require about 2000 to 2600 calories per day.[4] Dietary guidance for many older adults focuses on meeting nutrient recommendations while simultaneously reducing calories to maintain a healthy weight.

Carbohydrates and fiber
Carbohydrate requirements should be met with nutritious whole grains, fruits, and vegetables that are high in fiber. Limiting processed foods and sugar intake is also good dietary practice because foods that are high in added sugar are low in nutrients, high in calories, and replace more nutritious options.

More than 80% of Americans fail to eat the recommended amounts of vegetables and fruit.[4] Because intake of fruits, vegetables, and whole unprocessed grains is low in the typical American diet, fiber intake is also consistently below the recommended levels.[9] Chronic constipation in older adults affects approximately 50% of nursing home residents.[10] Older adults who consume a high-fiber diet will lower their risk of constipation. To reduce adverse effects, foods high in dietary fiber should be added slowly and fluid intake increased.[10] Many fiber-rich foods delay gastric emptying, resulting in the sensation of fullness, which although beneficial for weight loss, can be a problem for frail and underweight older adults struggling to consume adequate calories and meet nutritional requirements.

Fat
Older adults should choose dietary fats in similar distributions to those recommended for younger adults, including aiming for 5% to 6% of total calories from saturated fats and eliminating *trans* fats as much as possible.[11] However, fat is a valuable source of concentrated energy for frail and underweight older adults struggling to maintain a healthy body weight. In addition, dietary fat provides a necessary source of essential fatty acids, which may have the potential to prevent and reduce comorbidities and lower mortality.[12] Omega-3 fatty acids, in particular, may have benefits for reducing the risk of cognitive declines potentially treating age-related memory disorders, and also for maintaining muscle performance and immune function.[6,12] Dietary patterns that are predominantly plant-based and rich in healthy fats, such as the Mediterranean and the Mediterranean-DASH Intervention for Neurodegenerative Delay (MIND) diets are associated with the preservation of brain health including slower rates of cognitive decline, lower cognitive impairment, and reduced risk of dementia and Alzheimer disease.[13–16]

Protein

Nutrition guidance for older adults emphasizes adequate high-quality dietary protein to meet the metabolic and physiologic needs and prevent age-related loss of lean muscle mass that commonly accompanies aging. Some experts think that the current protein recommendation (0.8 g/kg body weight/d)[17] may not be adequate even as a minimum level for older adults[18] and recommend moderate increases in protein intake to enhance muscle protein metabolism and provide a mechanism for reducing progressive muscle loss.[19] Healthy older adults should aim to consume 1.2 to 2.0 g/kg body weight, which is significantly higher than the recommended dietary allowance (RDA).[20] The average intake of protein foods is lower for individuals aged 71 years and older compared with adults aged 60 through 70 years, and about 50% of women and 30% of men aged 71 years and older fall short of protein food recommendations.[4] Meeting protein recommendations may be challenging for older adults, especially for those with reduced appetite, functional and social limitations, and economic hardship. An even distribution of protein-rich foods throughout the day is suggested to help older adults consume adequate dietary protein. Including more protein-rich plant foods is beneficial in this group to help meet protein requirements and provide additional health benefits from dietary fiber, antioxidants, and phytochemicals while lowering dietary saturated fat and cholesterol.[21] In addition, older adults who followed a vegan diet experienced a 58% decrease in the number of prescribed medications, compared with those who followed a nonvegetarian diet.[22]

Fluids

Dehydration is the most common fluid and electrolyte disturbance in older adults and commonly occurs among institutionalized elderly (**Box 2**).[23]

Micronutrients: vitamins and minerals

Age-related changes in food intake, nutrient absorption, and metabolism can contribute to higher dietary requirements for many vitamins and minerals. Recommended intakes of vitamins and minerals for older adults take into consideration the variability in requirements and individual health status among this age group by offering recommendations for those aged 51 to 70 years and 70 years and older.[24] Although chronologic age is used as a cutoff for the Dietary Reference Intakes, actual nutrient requirements may be wide ranging in the older adult population.

Vitamin B$_{12}$. Vitamin B$_{12}$ deficiency characterized by neurologic abnormalities, including cognitive decline, peripheral neuropathy, decreased muscle strength, and functional disability[25] is estimated to be present in 1 in 8 older adults.[26] In institutionalized elderly residents, the prevalence of vitamin B$_{12}$ deficiency could be as high as 35%.[27] The ability to absorb vitamin B$_{12}$ decreases with age due to decreased gastric acid, lack of intrinsic factor, and atrophic gastritis with accompanying small bowel

---

Box 2
Hydration examples for older adults

- Water, unsweetened beverages, 100% fruit or vegetable juice, low-fat or fat-free milk, or unsweetened fortified plant milks
- Foods that have high water content: fruits, vegetables, and soups contribute to total fluid intake while helping to achieve food group recommendations
- Beverages that have added sugar and alcoholic beverages should be limited

bacterial overgrowth.[28] Older adults are encouraged to meet the recommendations for protein foods, a common source of vitamin B_{12}, and include foods fortified with vitamin B_{12} such as breakfast cereals in a healthy eating pattern.[4] As a result of gastric changes, it may be easier for older adults to absorb synthetic vitamin B_{12} from supplements and fortified foods than the B_{12} naturally present in foods.[29,30] Intranasal, sublingual, or intramuscular injections are indicated for those who lack the ability to absorb sufficient dietary or oral vitamin B_{12} supplements.

Vitamin D. Vitamin D facilitates calcium absorption from the gut, decreases the release of calcium from the kidneys, and increases calcium uptake in the bones. Vitamin D insufficiency and deficiency are common in the older population resulting from low dietary intake, limited sunlight exposure, and decreased skin synthesis and renal production of vitamin D.[31] Older adults who are deficient in vitamin D are at higher risk for osteomalacia, osteoporosis, and muscle weakness, which can lead to declines in mobility, physical performance and function, hip fractures, diabetes, cancer, heart disease, arthritis, depression, cognitive decline, and overall poor health.[32] Low-fat dairy products are good sources of calcium, vitamin D, and protein and are low in calories and fat, making them a good food choice for older adults. It can be challenging for older adults to consume the recommended amount of vitamin D from food alone; therefore, calcium and vitamin D supplementation may be needed in this population.[33]

Sodium. Ninety-four percent of older males and 72% of older females exceed the recommended daily limit of 2300 mg sodium.[4] Approximately 70% of the sodium in the typical American diet comes from processed, packaged, and restaurant foods, with almost 50% of the sodium in the US diet from mixed dishes (**Box 3**), foods commonly consumed by older adults.[34]

There is strong evidence of a dose-response effect of sodium reduction on blood pressure and that reducing dietary sodium lowers the risk of cardiovascular disease and stroke.[35,36] Older adults with hypertension can follow the Dietary Approaches to Stop Hypertension (DASH) dietary plan (**Box 4**).

The DASH diet is lower in sodium than the typical American diet and is also low in saturated fats while rich in potassium, calcium, magnesium, dietary fiber, and protein.[37] Dietary intake in older adults who are prescribed a low-sodium diet should be monitored regularly because although the sodium restriction has been shown to lower blood pressure, it may contribute to a bland diet, decrease food intake, and negatively affect nutritional status.

Antioxidants. Diets high in antioxidant-rich foods such as natural, unprocessed fruits and vegetables have been associated with many health benefits including a lower

---

Box 3
High-sodium mixed dishes commonly consumed by older Americans

- Sandwiches
- Pasta
- Grain dishes
- Pizza
- Meat, poultry, seafood dishes
- Soups

Box 4
The dietary approaches to stop hypertension diet

- High in vegetables, fruits, low-fat dairy products, whole grains, poultry, fish, beans, and nuts
- Low in sweets, sugar-sweetened beverages, and red meats

---

incidence of cardiovascular disease, age-related macular degeneration, diabetes, and cancer and also provide protection against dementia and other cognitive deteriorations common in aging.[38]

To reduce oxidative stress and inflammation, many experts recommend that older adults follow eating patterns that emphasize a plant-based diet and unprocessed foods. The MIND diet (**Box 5**) is a neuroprotective dietary pattern aimed specifically at protecting the brain and reducing dementia and declines in brain health associated with age.[39]

Research on the MIND diet in older adults has encouraging findings for those seeking to preserve brain health, slow cognitive decline, and reduce the risk of Alzheimer dementia with aging.[40–42] Older adults should aim to boost their food sources of antioxidants and use dietary supplements with medical supervision.

Alcohol

High quantities of alcohol intake can displace necessary nutrients, decrease appetite, alter taste perception, and interfere with the absorption, utilization, and nutritional balance in older adults who may have difficulty meeting nutritional recommendations and are at risk for malnutrition.[43,44] Nutritional guidance should help older adults move toward a healthy dietary pattern and minimize risks associated with alcohol consumption by limiting intake to 2 drinks or less per day for men and 1 drink or less per day for women.[4]

Nutritional and Dietary Supplements

Older adults use dietary supplements for overall wellness, for prevention or treatment of specific health conditions, for pain reduction, and to supplement conventional medical treatments. Seventy percent of older adults take 1 or more dietary supplements, and almost one-third take more than 4 supplements.[45] The most commonly used products are multivitamin/multimineral supplements, vitamin D, and omega-3 fatty acids.[45] Many adults, however, do not discuss their supplement use with a health care provider because they do not think of dietary supplements as medications. Dietary supplements have the potential to be beneficial, but if misused can be harmful to health. To the extent possible, older adults should aim to get their required nutrients from food as part of a healthy calorically balanced diet rather than from dietary

---

Box 5
Mediterranean-dietary approaches to stop hypertension intervention for neurodegenerative delay diet

- Encourages minimally processed plant foods such as vegetables, specifically green leafy vegetables, berries, nuts, olives and olive oil, whole grains, beans, fish, and poultry
- Limits foods from animal sources and foods high in saturated fat including butter and margarine, cheese, red meat, fried foods, pastries, sweets, processed desserts, and wine (<1 glass daily)

---

supplements.[28] Many older people find it difficult to eat enough nutrient-dense foods to meet their needs, so nutrient supplementation may be indicated to prevent deficiency or insufficiency and maintain health and body weight.

Factors that Affect Diet and Food Intake in Older Adults

Food provides more than just nourishment for all people, especially with advancing age. Meals contribute to a sense of security, add meaning and structure to the day, provide an opportunity for socialization, and boost psychological well-being. Health, social, psychological, physical, economic, and behavioral factors influence food intake (**Box 6**). Accessibility and preferences make the task of maximizing nutrition in older adults complicated.

Physical limitations and reduced functional status can make the simple tasks of shopping and cooking overwhelming, leading to progressive worsening of nutritional status, which further impairs health and well-being.

Clinical Nutrition Considerations for Older Adults

For most older adults aging is a continuum of deteriorating health and functionality, from independence to worsening disability, dependency, and disease. Nutritional status has a significant and direct impact on the progression and severity of disease. Disability of old age is commonly associated with age-dependent conditions that have nutritional implications such as coronary artery disease, diabetes, gastrointestinal conditions, and dementia, which are common causes of death. Careful analysis of all underlying diseases and conditions and appropriate individualized medical nutrition therapy (MNT), defined as *"nutritional diagnostic, therapy, and counseling services for the purpose of disease management which are furnished by a registered dietitian or nutrition professional..."* is crucial to the successful nutritional management of older adults.[46]

Up to half of older adults are malnourished or at risk of becoming malnourished.[47] Early identification of nutritional risks and malnutrition in older adults can be accomplished quickly and reliably by members of the interprofessional health care team using nutrition screening and assessment tools such as the Malnutrition Screening Tool,[48] Mini Nutritional Assessment (short form for elderly),[49] or the Subjective Global Assessment.[50–53] A comprehensive nutrition assessment that includes anthropometric, biochemical, clinical, neurologic, social, and dietary parameters is indicated when a potential risk has been identified. A nutrition-focused physical examination should be used when assessing the nutritional status of frail older adults and those with concurrent disability and medical conditions.[43] The Malnutrition Quality Improvement Initiative (MQII) is an evidence-based resource for interdisciplinary health care professionals to promote optimal nutrition standards of care and eliminate malnutrition. The MQII uses food insecurity as a hunger vital sign along with nutrition risk.[54]

Box 6
Significant nutritional influences

- Dietary behaviors and nutritional well-being:
  - Food security, education, finances, geographic location, literacy, and language
- Food choices and preparation methods:
  - Ethnic, cultural, religious beliefs, and long-standing food-related behaviors
- Ability to purchase wholesome foods:
  - Community-dwelling, food deserts, dependency on transportation, and limited finances

A patient requires further evaluation for malnutrition when 2 of the 6 characteristics (**Box 7**) are present.[44,46,47]

Malnourished older adults are at higher risk for infection and disease; poorer outcomes after traumatic injury; frailty; pressure ulcers; immune suppression; complications after surgery; longer, more expensive hospital stays; hospital readmission; and death.[47,48,51] Older adults should routinely be screened for food insecurity and other health disparities linked to malnutrition, which can worsen patient health and chronic illness and burden the health care system.[54]

An increasing number of older adults have overweight (body mass index [BMI] 25–30) or obesity (BMI >30) posing unprecedented medical challenges.[4] The prevalence of obesity among men and women aged 60 years is almost 43%.[55] Preventing additional weight gain and achieving a sustainable healthy weight by following a healthy dietary pattern and adopting an active lifestyle at any age supports healthy aging. Sarcopenia, the loss of skeletal muscle mass and function, affects up to 33% of community-dwelling older adults, with a higher prevalence in frail elders in long-term care and acute care settings. Conditions such as malnutrition, sarcopenia, and frailty are frequently undiagnosed and could be mitigated with early identification and intervention.[53,56] Sarcopenic obesity, the coexistence of obesity and sarcopenia, results from metabolic changes associated with a sedentary lifestyle, derangements in adipose tissue, and acute and chronic diseases.[57] Sarcopenic obesity contributes to worsening of health status, poor health outcomes, and increased frailty, disability, and physical dependency of older adults.[4–6,53] The simultaneous occurrence of both undernutrition and overnutrition in the same person is cause for concern and are important red flags to monitor for malnutrition.[7] Screening for dietary inadequacies, malnutrition, and food security should be included as part of routine nutrition evaluation for all older adults with risk factors including those who are frail, undernourished, overweight, or obese.[56,57] Optimizing nutritional intake, in particular adequate high-quality protein and antioxidants, is a nutritional priority for older adults with sarcopenia and sarcopenic obesity. Interventions that combine physical exercise, specifically progressive resistance strength training, with dietary strategies can reduce sarcopenia in older adults.[58]

As health declines, the need to individualize MNT and dietary recommendations becomes increasingly important, especially in the presence of multiple disease conditions. Nutrition intervention approaches and MNT should be interprofessional in nature and designed to meet the unique challenges of this population. Older adults are often placed on medically restrictive diets, which can become unpalatable and unenjoyable, thus worsening food intake and nutritional status. Dietary interventions for older adults should maximize medical treatment, respect aging body systems, preserve quality of life, and support overall well-being. Dietary prescriptions should be

---

Box 7
Clinical characteristics of malnutrition

- Inadequate energy intake
- Unintentional weight loss
- Loss of muscle mass
- Loss of subcutaneous fat
- Fluid accumulation (can disguise weight loss)
- Reduced functional status measured by handgrip strength

liberalized to the extent possible to promote healthy food intake and minimize unde-sirable weight loss and malnutrition.[47]

Older adults who can no longer perform the nutrition-related activites of daily living (ADLs) and instrumental activities of daily living (IADLs) such as feeding themselves and shopping and preparing foods are at risk for poor nutritional status. Anorexia of aging can result from a combination of physiologic, social, and pathologic conditions and may lead to protein-energy malnutrition and weight loss.[10] Polypharmacy is another potential factor that can impact nutritional status in older adults. Over-the-counter and prescription medication use should be regularly evaluated for potential side effects and drug-nutrient interactions.

End-of-Life Nutrition and Hydration Considerations

Near the end of life, patients often do not consume adequate calories and fluids to meet their needs. and older adults are vulnerable to poor decision making, abuse, and neglect. Food is considered to be part of palliative care that is necessary until death, and the expression "food first" continues to apply into old age if the person is able to eat. When a person is unable to eat enough to maintain body weight, artificial nutrition and hydration may be used to supplement or replace oral intake; however, there are many considerations regarding feeding and hydration in patients with organ failure.[59] Appropriate and compassionate end-of-life care, includes the attention to nutrition and hydration, and should be decided and documented when the older adult is able to soundly communicate their wishes if possible.

Nutrition Programs for Older Adults: Promoting Nutrition and Healthy Lifestyles for Older Adults

Eighty-five percent of noninstitutionalized older adults have at least 1 chronic health condition that could be improved with proper nutrition.[60] Sixty-six percent of all health care dollars in the United States are spent on managing chronic conditions in older adults.[2] Enabling older adults to stay at home and in their communities helps preserve a higher quality of life, reduce long-term health care costs, and maintain their indepen-dence and ties to family and friends. Participation in food and nutrition programs can improve dietary quality and health indicators for older adults. Federal food and nutri-tion assistance programs are a critical source of nutrition support for many older adults. Older adults have access to a variety of government resources to support a healthy dietary pattern as part of overall healthy aging. Professionals working with older Americans can use these resources to better support access to healthy, safe,

---

Box 8
Nutrition programs for older adults[4]

- Congregate Nutrition Services
- SNAP
- Commodity Supplemental Food Programs
- Home-Delivered Nutrition Services
- Child and Adult Care Food Program
- Seniors Farmers Market Nutrition Program

https://www.dietaryguidelines.gov/sites/default/files/2020-12/Dietary_Guidelines_for_Americans_2020-2025.pdf.

Abbreviation: SNAP, Supplemental Nutrition Assistance Program.

and affordable food choices. There are several programs (**Box 8**) intended to fight hunger that service older adults, and nutrition programs aimed at promoting health in older adults should be integrated into the overall health care plan.

SUMMARY

Good nutrition is a fundamental component of healthy aging. It can be difficult for older adults to meet their nutritional needs because of their increased requirements for some nutrients, lower energy needs, and numerous health and lifestyle barriers to adequate food intake. The maintenance of good health for the growing population of older adults requires approaches that recognize multiple levels of influence on the individual medical, social, cultural, environmental, organizational, and personal factors. Older adults should be encouraged to consume a variety of nutrient-dense foods, and supplementation should be considered when dietary intake is inadequate. Nutrition services and programs are vital to making a positive impact in the lives of older adults. Health care providers have opportunities to help older adults promote and maintain their health and enjoy a good quality of life by developing thoughtful strategic nutrition care plans.

CLINICS CARE POINTS

- Old age is associated with increased burden of poor health, polypharmacy, reduced socialization, and limited functional ability, which can contribute to poor nutritional status; therefore high-quality dietary intake is essential for promoting well-being, maintenance of functional status, and preventing malnutrition as well as acute and chronic comorbidities.

- Older adults may have reduced calorie requirements and therefore should carefully choose foods that are nutritionally dense such as fresh and minimally processed vegetables and fruits, whole grains, and high-quality protein-rich foods while limiting sugar, saturated fat, sodium, and processed foods.

- Older adults should aim to meet their nutritional needs with healthy foods and use dietary supplements with guidance from health care providers.

- Older adults should be regularly screened for common nutrition-related conditions such as sarcopenic obesity, malnutrition, frailty, dehydration, and constipation.

- Medically restrictive diets are important for the nutritional management of many conditions but should be implemented with caution because limitations could contribute to decreased food intake and negatively affect nutritional status.

- The goal for nutritional health in adults at every age should be to preserve physical and mental well-being and maintain a high quality of life.

DISCLOSURE

M. Bernstein receives a portion of author royalties from Jones and Bartlett Learning in association with the publication of Nutrition, Discovering Nutrition, Nutrition for Older Adults, Nutrition Assessment Clinical and Research Applications, and Nutrition Across Life Stages.

REFERENCES

1. 2019 Profile of Older Americans. Administration for Community Living and Administration on Aging. 2021. Available at: https://acl.gov/sites/default/files/Aging%

20and%20Disability%20in%20America/2020ProfileOlderAmericans.Final_.pdf. Accessed January 4, 2022.

2. Fact sheet: aging in the United States 2019. Population Reference Bureau Web site. Available at: https://www.prb.org/resources/fact-sheet-aging-in-the-united-states/. Accessed February 28, 2022.

3. Healthy people 2030. Older Adults. U.S. Department of Health and Human Services. Office of Disease Prevention and Health Promotion Web site. Available at: https://health.gov/healthypeople/objectives-and-data/browse-objectives/older-adults. Accessed March 3, 2023.

4. Dietary Guidelines for Americans, 2020-2025. 9th edition. U.S. Department of Agriculture and U.S. Department of Health and Human Services Web site. DietaryGuidelines.gov; 2020. Accessed March 3, 2023.

5. Long T, Zhang K, Chen Y, et al. Trends in diet quality among older US Adults From 2001 to 2018. JAMA Netw Open 2022;5(3):e221880.

6. Plant–Based Diets and Longevity. American College of Lifestyle Medicine Web site. Available at: https://lifestyle-medicine.foleon.com/wfpb-nutrition/longevity/key-points-for-practitioners/. Accessed March 3, 2023.

7. MYPlate. Older Adults. USDA Web site. Available at: https://www.myplate.gov/life-stages/older-adults. Accessed March 3, 2023.

8. Robinson M, Mogensen K, Casey J, et al. The Relationship Among Obesity, Nutritional Status, and Mortality in the Critically Ill. Crit Care Med 2015;43(1):87–100.

9. Quagliani D, Felt-Gunderson P. Closing America's fiber intake gap. Am J Lifestyle Med 2017;11(1):80–5.

10. Mounsey A MD, Raleigh M, et al. Management of constipation in older adults. Am Fam Physician 2015;92(6):500–4. Available at: https://www.clinicalkey.es/playcontent/1-s2.0-S0002838X15302641.

11. Saturated Fat. American Heart Association Web site. Available at: https://www.heart.org/en/healthy-living/healthy-eating/eat-smart/fats/saturated-fats#:~:text=AHA%20Recommendation,of%20saturated%20fat%20per%20day. Accessed March 3, 2023.

12. Molfino A, Gioia G, Rossi Fanelli F, et al. The role for dietary omega-3 fatty acids supplementation in older adults. Nutrients 2014;6(10):4058–72.

13. Flanagan E, Lamport D, Brennan L, et al. Nutrition and the ageing brain: Moving towards clinical applications. Ageing Res Rev 2020;62:101079.

14. Liu Y, Gao X, Na M, et al. Dietary pattern, diet quality, and dementia: a systematic review and meta-analysis of prospective cohort studies. J Alzheimer's Dis 2020; 78(1):151–218.

15. Barbaresko J, Lellmann AW, Schmidt A, et al. Dietary factors and neurodegenerative disorders: an umbrella review of meta-analyses of prospective studies. Adv Nutr (Bethesda, Md 2020;11(5):1161–73.

16. Moradi S, Moloudi J, Moradinazar M, et al. Adherence to Healthy Diet Can Delay Alzheimer's diseases development: a systematic review and meta-analysis. Prev Nutr Food Sci 2020;25(4):325–37.

17. Institute of Medicine. Protein and amino acids. The National Academies Press; 2005. p. 589.

18. Volpi E, Campbell WW, Dwyer JT, et al. Is the optimal level of protein intake for older adults greater than the recommended dietary allowance? Journals Gerontology Ser A, Biol Sci Med Sci 2013;68(6):677–81.

19. Paddon-Jones D, Rasmussen B. Dietary protein recommendations and the prevention of sarcopenia. Curr Opin Clin Nutr Metab Care 2009;12(1):86–90.

20. Baum JI, Kim I, Wolfe RR. Protein consumption and the elderly: what is the optimal level of intake? Nutrients 2016;8(6):359.
21. Kahleova H, Levin S, Barnard ND. Plant-based diets for healthy aging. J Am Coll Nutr 2021;40(5):478–9.
22. Dos Santos H, Gaio J, Durisic A, et al. The polypharma study: association between diet and amount of prescription drugs among seniors. American journal of lifestyle medicine 2021;155982762110488. https://doi.org/10.1177/15598276211048812.
23. Bruno C, Collier A, Holyday M, et al. Interventions to Improve Hydration in Older Adults: A Systematic Review and Meta-Analysis. Nutrients 2021;13(10):3640.
24. Dietary reference intakes: vitamins. Institute of Medicine Web site. Available at: https://www.nationalacademies.org/hmd/~/media/Files/Activity%20Files/Nutrition/DRIs/DRI_Vitamins.pdf. Accessed February 27, 2022.
25. Oberlin BS, Tangney CC, Gustashaw KAR, et al. Vitamin B12 Deficiency in Relation to Functional Disabilities. Nutrients 2013;5(11):4462–75.
26. Laird EJ, O'Halloran AM, Carey D, et al. Voluntary fortification is ineffective to maintain the vitamin B12 and folate status of older Irish adults: evidence from the Irish Longitudinal Study on Ageing (TILDA). Br J Nutr 2018;120(1):111–20.
27. Wong CW, Ip CY, Leung CP, et al. Vitamin B12 deficiency in the institutionalized elderly: A regional study. Exp Gerontol 2015;69:221–5.
28. Bernstein M, Munoz N. Position of the Academy of Nutrition and Dietetics: Food and Nutrition for Older Adults: Promoting Health and Wellness. J Acad Nutr Diet 2012;112(8):1255–77. Available at: https://agris.fao.org/agris-search/search.do?recordID=US201500079814.
29. Baik HW, Russell RM. Vitamin B12 deficiency in the elderly. Annu Rev Nutr 1999;19(1):357–77.
30. Porter KM, Hoey L, Hughes CF, et al. Associations of atrophic gastritis and proton-pump inhibitor drug use with vitamin B-12 status, and the impact of fortified foods, in older adults. Am J Clin Nutr 2021;114(4):1286–94.
31. Dietary reference intakes for calcium and vitamin D. Institute of medicine of the national academies web site. 2010. Available at: http://www.nationalacademies.org/hmd/Reports/2010/Dietary-Reference-Intakes-for-Calcium-and-Vitamin-D/DRI-Values.aspx. Accessed February 27, 2022.
32. Meehan M, Penckofer S. The role of vitamin D in the aging adult. J Aging Gerontol 2014;2(2):60–71.
33. Sahni S, Mangano KM, Kiel DP, et al. Dairy intake is protective against bone loss in older vitamin d supplement users: the framingham study. J Nutr 2017;147(4):645–52.
34. Harnack L, Cogswell M, Shikany J, et al. Sources of Sodium in US Adults From 3 Geographic Regions. Circulation (New York, N.Y.) 2017;135(19):1775–83.
35. Cogswell ME, Mugavero K, Bowman BA, et al. Dietary sodium and cardiovascular disease risk — measurement matters. New Engl J Med 2016;375(6):580–6.
36. Mozaffarian D, Fahimi S, Singh GM, et al. Global Burden of Diseases Nutrition and Chronic Diseases Expert Group. Global sodium consumption and death from cardiovascular causes. N Engl J Med 2014;371(7):624–34.
37. Description of the DASH eating plan. . National Heart, Lung, and Blood Institute Web site. Available at: http://www.nhlbi.nih.gov/health/health-topics/topics/dash. Accessed February 27, 2022.
38. Yeh T, Yuan C, Ascherio A, et al. Long-term dietary flavonoid intake and subjective cognitive decline in US men and women. Neurology 2021;97(10):e1041–56.

39. van den Brink AC, Brouwer-Brolsma EM, Berendsen AAM, et al. The Mediterranean, Dietary Approaches to Stop Hypertension (DASH), and Mediterranean-DASH Intervention for Neurodegenerative Delay (MIND) diets are associated with less cognitive decline and a lower risk of Alzheimer's Disease-A Review. Adv Nutr 2019;10(6):1040–65.

40. Morris MC, Tangney CC, Wang Y, et al. MIND diet associated with reduced incidence of Alzheimer's disease. Alzheimer's Demen 2015;11(9):1007–14.

41. Morris MC, Tangney CC, Wang Y, et al. MIND diet slows cognitive decline with aging. Alzheimer's Demen 2015;11(9):1015–22.

42. Hosking DE, Eramudugolla R, Cherbuin N, et al. MIND not Mediterranean diet related to 12-year incidence of cognitive impairment in an Australian longitudinal cohort study. Alzheimer's Demen 2019;15(4):581–9.

43. Kuerbis Alexis, LCSW PhD, Sacco Paul, et al. Substance Abuse Among Older Adults. Clin Geriatr Med 2014;30(3):629–54.

44. Heuberger RA. Alcohol and the older adult: a comprehensive review. J Nutr Elder 2009;28(3):203–35.

45. Gahche JJ, Bailey RL, Potischman N, et al. Dietary supplement use was very high among older adults in the United States in 2011-2014. J Nutr 2017;147(10): 1968–76.

46. MNT versus nutrition education. eatrightPRO. Academy of nutrition and dietetics web site. 2006. Available at: https://www.eatrightpro.org/payment/coding-and-billing/mnt-vs-nutrition-education. Accessed March 13, 2022.

47. Malnutrition Quality Collaborative. National Blueprint: achieving quality malnutrition care for older adults. 2020 update. Avalere Health and Defeat Malnutrition Today; 2020.

48. Abbott Nutrition. Malnutrition Screening Tool (MST). Available at: https://static.abbottnutrition.com/cms-prod/abbottnutrition-2016.com/img/Malnutrition%20Screening%20Tool_FINAL_tcm1226-57900.pdf Web site. Accessed March 13, 2022.

49. Donini LM, Marrocco W, Marocco C, et al. Validity of the Self-Mini Nutritional Assessment (Self-MNA) for the Evaluation of Nutritional Risk. A Cross-Sectional Study Conducted in General Practice. J Nutr Health Aging 2018;22(1):44–52.

50. Duerksen DR, Laporte M, Jeejeebhoy K. Evaluation of nutrition status using the subjective global assessment: malnutrition, cachexia, and sarcopenia. Nutr Clin Pract 2021;36(5):942–56.

51. House M, Gwaltney C. Malnutrition screening and diagnosis tools: Implications for practice. Nutr Clin Pract 2022;37(1):12–22.

52. Malone A, Mogensen KM. Key approaches to diagnosing malnutrition in adults. Nutr Clin Pract 2022;37(1):23–34.

53. Dwyer JT, Gahche JJ, Weiler M, et al. Screening community-living older adults for protein energy malnutrition and frailty: update and next steps. J Community Health 2019;45(3):640–60.

54. MQii and the Nutrition Care Process. MQii Malnutrition Quality Improvement Initiative Web site. Updated 2021. Available at: https://malnutritionquality.org/. Accessed March 13, 2022.

55. Hales CM, Carroll MD, Fryar CD, et al. Prevalence of obesity and severe obesity among adults: United States, 2017-2018. Center for Disease Control and Prevention Web site; 2020. Accessed March 13, 2022. https://www.cdc.gov/nchs/products/databriefs/db360.htm.

56. Gahche JJ, Arensberg MB, Weiler M, et al. Opportunities for adding undernutrition and frailty screening measures in US National Surveys. Adv Nutr (Bethesda, Md 2021;12(6):2312–20.

57. Donini LM, Busetto L, Bischoff SC, et al. Definition and diagnostic criteria for sarcopenic obesity: ESPEN and EASO consensus statement. Obes facts 2022;1–15. https://doi.org/10.1159/000521241.

58. Naseeb MA, Volpe SL. Protein and exercise in the prevention of sarcopenia and aging. Nutr Res (New York, N.Y.) 2017;40:1–20.

59. Heuberger RA. Geriatric nutrition. Bernstein MA, McMahon K, editor. Jones and Bartlett. 2023. Nutrition Across Life Stages 3rd edition. P. 491-534

60. Supporting older patients with chronic conditions. National Institute on Aging Web site. 2022. Available at: https://www.nia.nih.gov/health/supporting-older-patients-chronic-conditions#:~:text=Approximately%2085%25%20of%20older%20adults,conditions%20is%20a%20real%20challenge.

Nutrition for the Athlete
A Foundation for Success

Gabriela Barreto, MS, RD, CDN, CSSD*

KEYWORDS

- Sports nutrition • Performance nutrition • Athlete • Endurance

KEY POINTS

- Athletes have a large energy requirement that should be met strategically to optimize performance and avoid low energy availability.
- The primary fuel source for athletes are carbohydrates. The amount needed is determined by the intensity and duration of training.
- Nutrient timing of proteins, carbohydrates, and fats are key to successfully restoring glycogen stores, repairing muscle and exercise-induced inflammation, and for recovery.
- Hydration needs are unique to other nutrient needs and require individualized attention.

INTRODUCTION

Nutrition for high-level athletes has become a crucial role in their performance, health, and ability to achieve success. Research on sports nutrition began in the 1960s and 1970s, looking at energy systems in sport and exercise.[1] Understanding an athlete's energy and nutrient needs sets the foundation for their nutrition plan. As an athlete's energy needs can often be double their resting metabolic rate (RMR), it is imperative that their nutrition plan covers their needs with adequate carbohydrates, protein, and fat.[2] This is to ensure optimal performance as well as avoid low energy availability (LEA), a state in which an athlete is not consuming enough calories to cover training and metabolism, leading to detriments to health and performance.[3]

Athletes produce energy for sport via three primary systems: phosphocreatine (PCr), anaerobic glycolysis, and aerobic system.[1,2,4] Athletes primarily use carbohydrates as a source of energy throughout the anaerobic and aerobic energy systems, and therefore, adequate carbohydrate intake is crucial.[2] Fat is also used as a source of energy when training is submaximal and long duration.[1,2,4] Although protein can be used for energy, its main role is to contribute to muscle protein synthesis (MPS) and muscle maintenance.

Staint Joseph's University, 245 Clinton Avenue, Brooklyn, NY 11205, USA
* Corresponding author.
E-mail address: nutritionbygabby@gmail.com

Physician Assist Clin 7 (2022) 727–740
https://doi.org/10.1016/j.cpha.2022.06.004
2405-7991/22/© 2022 Elsevier Inc. All rights reserved.

When providing care to athletes, creating a team approach to medical care and treatment will allow for more favorable outcomes. Nutrition recommendations are a vital part of the treatment of athletes. Screening for LEA, nutrient deficiencies, and disordered eating and monitoring and referrals to allied professionals are an integral part of patient care. This article explains the role of nutrition and the registered dietitian nutritionist (RDN) in an athlete's health and performance, emphasizing a collaborative approach to care.

BACKGROUND
Energy Pathways in Sport

There are three main pathways for the body to produce energy to sustain muscular contractions. The production of adenosine triphosphate (ATP) occurs via the anaerobic system, including PCr, and the breakdown of carbohydrates to lactic acid via glycolysis. The production of ATP also occurs through the aerobic system using carbohydrates and fats.[1,2] Although these systems may work concurrently, the degree to which each system dominates depends on the intensity, often expressed as a percentage of maximal oxygen consumption (Vo_{2max}) as well as the duration of training.[1,4] At lower intensities and percentage of Vo_{2max}, the body relies more heavily on the aerobic system, using fat and glucose as fuel.[1,2,4] At higher intensities and closer to one's Vo_{2max}, the body relies on the rapid production of ATP via anaerobic systems.[1,2,4] **Table 1** describes the predominant system based on exercise intensity and duration. Both are always being used, but the need for ATP and the availability of oxygen will determine which is more predominant.[1,2,4]

Weight lifters and sprinters can rapidly produce large power outputs at maximal effort.[1] Generation of ATP for maximal power output relies on anaerobic ATP production. The anaerobic system is generally predominant at a higher percentage of an athlete's Vo_{2max}, higher exercise intensity, and shorter duration.[1,2,4] The anaerobic system allows for a rapid production of ATP to produce powerful muscle outputs for a single bout of exercise.[1] The PCr system rapidly produces ATP for immediate energy, supplying ATP for 10 to 30 seconds of work.[1,4] After the first 10 seconds, ATP supplied by the PCr system rapidly declines by 50% to 85%.[1,4] This energy supply is short-lived due to small amounts of PCr stored in muscle.[2] The system can only replenish when the intensity of exercise declines or work ends.[4]

The anaerobic breakdown of carbohydrates to lactic acid and pyruvic acid occurs via glycolysis.[1,2,4] This system is predominant within the first 90 to 100 seconds of work at near maximal levels of one's maximal oxygen uptake (Vo_2).[1,2] Glucose is broken down from carbohydrate-rich foods and circulates in the blood or is stored as glycogen in the liver and skeletal muscle. In anaerobic glycolysis, one glucose molecule is oxidized into two pyruvic acid molecules.[2] This system lasts from 30 seconds to 2 minutes of maximal effort exercise.[1,4] This system is limited due to the

Table 1		
Energy System, Intensity and Duration[1,4]		
Energy System	**Exercise Intensity**	**Time**
Phosphocreatine system	High	~10 s
Anaerobic glycolysis	Moderate–high	~30 s–2 min
Aerobic	Low–moderate	~4 min and above

absence of oxygen, resulting in pyruvic acid being converted to lactic acid.[2] Lactic acid either produces hydrogen ions or dissociates into lactate.[2] As hydrogen molecules accumulate, the pH of muscle drops, enzyme activity decreases, and muscle fatigues.[1,2] This causes the body to decrease work output or stop activity to recover.[1] Lactate is more readily cleared from the muscle by either being taken up into the mitochondria, transported to other cells for oxidation, or being used to produce energy in the liver via the Cori cycle.[2] In the presence of oxygen, pyruvic acid can continue into aerobic glycolysis via the Krebs cycle.[2]

The aerobic system can provide a large supply of ATP via the Krebs cycle and the electron transport chain (ETC).[2] This system is predominant at lower intensities of exercise where submaximal levels of Vo_2 can be sustained at a steady state. However, studies have shown that the aerobic system can contribute to a degree at higher intensities.[1] During submaximal intensities, with the greater availability of oxygen, the body can better use fatty acids through beta-oxidation and electrons via the ETC as a primary source of ATP to sustain training.[2,4] One glucose molecule can be oxidized to produce ~32 ATP molecules, and one fat molecule can produce ~106 ATP molecules.[2] This system can provide an almost limitless supply of ATP via the Krebs cycle and the ETC as long as enough oxygen and nutrients are present.[2]

When fueling athletes, understanding their primary energy systems is essential when determining fueling needs. Endurance and ultra-endurance athletes, such as runners, cyclists, and triathletes, will rely mainly on aerobic glycolysis and fatty acid oxidation due to the long duration of their sport. On the contrary, a power athlete, such as a powerlifter, Olympic lifter, or sprinter, will rely on the PCr system or anaerobic glycolysis due to the short explosive nature of their sport. Athletes will use all three energy systems to varying degrees depending on the intensity and duration of training.

DISCUSSION
Setting a Sports Nutrition Foundation

Determining energy and macronutrient needs is most important and the foundation of an athlete's nutrition plan. Although sports nutrition marketing may highlight the benefits of supplements, most of the benefits of enhanced performance will come from a well-designed foundation. The athlete's performance pyramid seen in **Fig. 1** displays the importance of an adequate foundation in relation to performance-specific recommendations and supplements.

Determining Energy Needs

Athletes' energy needs are high to account for rigorous training and recovery needs. An athlete's RMR can often be half of their total energy needs.[2] In determining an athlete's needs, it is essential to ensure they have adequate energy availability to compete and train successfully. A goal in determining energy needs is to avoid LEA, which is defined as the energy left for metabolic processes after accounting for the energy used during training.[3] LEA can have numerous consequences on an athlete's health and performance.[3]

To determine energy needs, indirect calorimetry is a tool to measure an athlete's RMR.[2] These devices use measurements of oxygen consumed and carbon dioxide produced to determine energy use at rest.[2] An individual's RMR is based on numerous factors, including, but not limited to, age, gender, height, weight, and body composition. Depending on what anthropometric information is available, an estimated RMR can be calculated using the following equations:

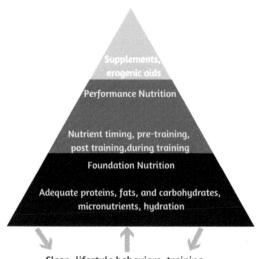

Fig. 1. Athletes performance pyramid.

Mifflin-St. Jeor

Men: RMR = (10 × wt [kg]) + (6.25 × ht [cm]) − (5 × age [y]) + 5
Women: RMR = (10 × wt [kg]) + (6.25 × ht [cm]) − (5 × age [y]) −161

Harris–Benedict

Men: RMR = 66 +(13.7 × wt [kg]) + (5 × ht [cm]) − (6.8 × age [y])
Women: RMR = 655 +(9.6 × wt [kg]) + (1.8 × ht [cm]) − (4.7 × age [y])

Cunningham equation (requires fat-free mass measurement [FFM])
RMR = 370 + (21.6 × FFM [kg])

The Cunningham equation is most accurate in predicting an athlete's RMR, though it requires a fat-free mass measurement that may not be available.[2] Harris–Benedict would be the next best equation to use for this population.[2] After determining an athlete's RMR, coefficients known as activity factors can be used to determine total daily energy expenditure (TDEE).[2] These activity factors (AF) correlate with the level of physical activity and are multiplied to determine an athlete's energy and overall nutrient needs (**Table 2**).

Table 2 Activity factors[5]	
Intensity and Frequency of Exercise	**AF**
Sedentary: little to no exercise	**1.2**
Light activity: light exercise 1–3x per week	1.375
Moderate activity: moderate exercise/sport 6–7x per week	1.55
Very active: hard exercise every day or 2x per day	1.725
Extra active: hard exercise 2x per day; training for an endurance event	1.9

Below is an example of determining the energy needs of an athlete.
Example of Athlete A (Mifflin-St. Jeor):
25 years, 61 kg female athlete, 170 cm. Plays professional soccer, trains 2x a day 4 to 5 days a week.
RMR= (10 × 61 kg) + (6.25 × 170) − (5 × 25) −161 = 1386 kcal.
TDEE = 1386 kcal × 1.9 AF = **> 2633 kcal**
In the above example, approximately 2630 calories would be meeting Athlete A's energy needs. Her metabolism is 1386 kcal and the energy she uses for training and activities of daily living is approximately 1245 kcal. If Athlete A was to consume 1900 calories, she would be experiencing LEA. To determine her energy availability in this scenario, the following equation is used:
Energy Availability = Energy Intake (kcal) − Energy expenditure during exercise (kcal)
= 1900 kcal − 1245 kcal.
= 655 kcal.
In this example, Athlete A's energy availability is only 655 kcal. This is the energy available to complete all her metabolic tasks and would be considered LEA. Adequate energy availability for optimal physiologic function is achieved at 45 cal/kg of fat-free mass per day, with disturbances being seen at less than 30 cal/kg of fat-free mass per day.[3,6] LEA in athletes can be categorized as intentional via disordered eating or unintentional due to high activity levels and inadequate intake.[3,6] Symptoms of LEA range from menstrual dysfunction to decreased bone mineral density and decreased performance as well as gastrointestinal, cardiac, phycological, endocrine, and metabolic dysfunction.[3,6] The related conditions to LEA, the Female Athlete Triad and Relative Energy Deficiency in Sport, will be discussed in the companion article titled, Nutrition for the Athlete: Beyond the Basics.

Body composition can play a role in an athlete's sport. Athletes may strive to alter their body composition by gaining muscle to produce more power and strength. In some sports organizations, athletes may need to maintain a specific weight and body fat percentage for a specific position. This is to ensure the fairness of competition. Weight-class athletes such as those in combat sport, powerlifters, and Olympic weightlifters must make a specific weight to compete. Several tactics and strategies are used during longitudinal and acute weight loss. A review by Reale and colleagues on acute weight loss strategies for combat sport athletes provides an in-depth review of evidence-based practices.[7]

Performance indicators may be impacted by body composition. A study on soccer players found that a higher body fat mass was detrimental to speed.[8] In volleyball players, a study has shown that lower body fat and higher muscle mass contributed positively to vertical jump scores.[9] Contrarily, athletes with a low body mass index and inappropriate body composition can experience disturbed athletic performance.[10] Although there are noted advantages to being at a lower body fat percentage, no standard body fat percentage and muscle mass percentage have been identified for optimal performance. In addition, athletes may struggle with body image, disordered eating, and LEA.[3,6] It is important to emphasize performance markers, meeting energy needs, and health before body composition.

As noted, weight loss or weight gain may be helpful in an athlete's success in sport. This should be achieved with the assistance of an RDN who specializes in sports to ensure the athlete is getting adequate nutrition while reaching their body composition goals. Although low-carbohydrate diets are popular in the general weight loss population, eliminating carbohydrate-rich foods, even when pursuing weight loss, is not advised and will be detrimental to athletic performance.

Carbohydrates

In the 1920s, carbohydrates became recognized as a primary fuel source.[11] Carbohydrates via blood glucose and muscle glycogen are the primary source of energy and fuel for athletic performance at intensities greater than 60% Vo_{2max}.[2,11] The body stores carbohydrates in the form of glycogen, which break down into glucose via glycolysis to provide energy for working organs and muscles. The two main sites for glycogen storage are the liver and muscles.[11,12] Dependent on diet, the liver stores greater than 80 g glycogen which can supply muscle and circulating blood, containing about 4 g glucose, during training. Muscle, on average, contains 500 g of glycogen.[11] In the muscles, glycogen is readily available to be broken down into glucose and used for the exercising muscle to generate ATP. Consuming carbohydrates before training allows for glucose to be readily available in circulating blood for use.[11,12]

Carbohydrate needs are specific to the duration and intensity of the sport and should be adjusted to match training needs. The range set for carbohydrate needs is 3 to 12 g/kg and depends on the length and intensity of the training or sport.[13] For example, an athlete participating in moderate to high-intensity training for 2 to 3 hours a day will require 6 to 10 g/kg of carbohydrates per day.[12] **Box 1** provides the recommended carbohydrate needs dependent on the time and intensity of exercise. These should be strategically spaced throughout the day, with carbohydrates considered pretraining, during, and posttraining.[2,12,13] The timing and distribution of carbohydrates are important for fueling and recovering from athletic performance.[2,12,13]

Dietary interventions and training status influence glycogen storage, usage, and availability.[12] The availability of glycogen stores will significantly impact an athlete's performance, and therefore, its refueling and recovery are essential.[12] Pretraining carbohydrate intake ensures the availability of adequate carbohydrates immediately for training.[11] Suboptimal carbohydrate stores are available in a fasted state and therefore fasted training is unsupported and not recommended.[12] To ensure carbohydrates are available for use, research shows that consuming carbohydrates less than 60 g before training provides elevated blood glucose levels for training.[12] The recommended amount of carbohydrate before training is 1 to 4 g/kg of body mass, ranging from 75 to 300 g for a 75 kg athlete.[13] In practice, the high end of carbohydrates can be challenging for an athlete to reach due to the volume of food and the ability of the gut to absorb and perform. Working with a sports dietitian, an athlete can learn how to distribute these needs reasonably within an individualized plan.

An important consideration is the form and type of carbohydrates. Pretraining, low-fiber carbohydrate sources are recommended.[13] Examples of such foods are melon fruits, banana, pineapple, white bread with jelly, dried fruit, and fig bars. **Table 3** provides a list of common carbohydrate foods for athletes. Lower fiber content will allow for faster absorption. Although the glycemic index of foods has been researched on whether there is a benefit between high versus low-glycemic carbohydrate pretraining, the overall evidence remains equivocal.[12–15]

Box 1 Carbohydrates Needs for Athletes	
Intensity	**Carbohydrate Needs**
Low Intensity (i.e. skills training, drills)	3-5 g/kg/day
Moderate Intensity (~1 hour training per day)	5-7 g/kg/day
High Intensity (i.e. endurance training, 1-3 hours training per day)	6-10 g/kg/day
Very High Intensity (>4-5 hours training per day)	8-12 g/kg/day

Table 3
Carbohydrate-rich foods for athletes

Carbohydrate Source	Grams of Carbohydrates
Pasta, 1 cup spaghetti	67 g
Potato, 1 large (3" −4.25" diameter)	65 g
Fig bars, 1 oz	20 g
Bagel	50 g
Black beans, 1 cup	45 g
Orange, 1 cup	27 g
Grapes, 1 cup	15 g
Granola bar	20 g
Banana, 1 medium	27 g
Rice, 1 cup	53 g
Pineapple, 1 cup	22 g

Adapted from USDA National Nutrient Database for Standard Reference Legacy.[16]

Prolonged high-intensity training exceeding 60 minutes, including stop-and-go sports, may benefit from carbohydrate consumption during training.[13] This provides adequate carbohydrates to prevent a dip in blood sugar and optimize performance as muscle glycogen and liver stores deplete. Sustained high-intensity training for 45 to 75 minutes may benefit from small amounts of carbohydrate from a sports drink or mouth rinse.[13] Training 1 to 2.5 hours will benefit from 30 to 60 g/h of carbohydrates in the form of sports beverages or sports performance food products.[13] Endurance training exceeding 2.5 hours may require up to 90 g/h, and multiple carbohydrate sources are recommended.[13]

The source and type of carbohydrate are also important for absorbing and delivering glucose to blood, liver, and muscle, particularly in endurance sports. Once broken down, monosaccharides are taken up by transporters in the gut. There are multiple transporters which transport specific monosaccharides into the bloodstream, as detailed in **Table 4**. Gastrointestinal issue may arise if a specific transporter becomes oversaturated.[12] This includes gastric emptying, absorption of carbohydrate and fluid, and potential for gastrointestinal distress.[12] This can impact the availability of glucose for training and glycogen resynthesis.[12] Multiple transportable carbohydrates aid in providing both glucose and fructose to prevent over saturation of these transporters to enhance absorption and alleviate gastric concerns.[12] Studies have shown that mixed carbohydrate sources of glucose + fructose or maltodextrin + fructose enhance absorption and fluid delivery, decrease gastrointestinal distress, and improve gastric emptying versus glucose alone.[12]

Posttraining, the ability to absorb, transport, and synthesize glycogen, is enhanced.[17] Muscle cells are sensitive to nutrients immediately following training. Therefore, consuming a carbohydrate-rich posttraining snack or meal is vital for

Table 4
Carbohydrate transporters in the gut

Transporter	Carbohydrates Transported
Sodium/glucose cotransporter 1 (SGLT1)	Glucose and galactose
Glucose transporter 2 (GLUT2)	Glucose, fructose, and galactose
Glucose transporter 5 (GLUT5)	Fructose

muscle recovery and restoring muscle glycogen. To optimize glycogen stores, athletes should consume greater than 1 g/kg of carbohydrate every 2 hours in the first 4 hours posttraining.[17] This feeding should occur immediately within the first 2 hours following training. Protein consumption with low carbohydrate intake, 0.8 g/kg carbohydrate with 0.4 g/kg protein posttraining, can enhance glycogen repletion similarly to higher carbohydrate, 1.2 g/kg intake.[17]

Protein

Protein in skeletal muscle is constantly broken down by muscle protein breakdown and rebuilt by MPS. MPS is elevated for 24 hours posttraining, and therefore, the timing of protein and overall nutrition is important to maintain and build muscle mass.[18] Protein is most effective in eliciting MPS when consumed evenly in balanced meals and snacks and spaced throughout the day, starting at breakfast.[19] This has been noted when compared with consuming large amounts of protein distributed among two meals a day.[19]

To elicit MPS, studies have shown that at least 20 g of high-quality protein or 0.31 g protein/kg of body weight per meal or posttraining supplementation will stimulate MPS.[20–22] To stimulate MPS, it is imperative that adequate amino acids, specifically 2.5 g leucine, are available. Milk-based protein, such as whey protein isolate, is a favorable and effective source posttraining.[23] This is because of the amino acid pool found in whey protein.[23] Protein needs are higher in an athletic population, ranging from 1.2 to 2.0 g/kg per day.[2,18] This is because of the higher nutrient needs of athletes and the high rate of protein turnover. Protein intake before and during training may be helpful to athletes looking to increase muscle size.[18] Athletes still need to ensure adequate carbohydrates and fats for optimal performance, and excessive protein intake is not recommended.

Protein quality is of importance. Essential amino acid (EAA) content is critical in assessing a quality protein source to adequately stimulate MPS, specifically leucine content.[23] Animal-based proteins ranging from 20 to 25 g contain higher EAA content and will provide the leucine threshold needed for MPS.[24] As for plant-based protein, it can take 20 to 54 g to reach that same leucine threshold.[24] Although animal-based diets offer an advantage, a well-planned plant-based diet can meet an athlete's needs. **Table 5** provides the sources of protein and their leucine content.

Fat

Athletes must meet their fat needs and can do so with a well-balanced performance diet. The recommended amount of fat for athletes is 1 g/kg because the need for

Table 5	
Leucine content of protein foods	
Protein Source	**Leucine Content**
Swiss Cheese, 1 cup diced	3.9 g
Tofu, ½ cup	1.7 g
Turkey, 1 cup diced	2.8 g
Beef, 3 oz	2.5 g
Edamame, 1 cup	1.5 g
Peas, 1 cup	0.328 g
Milk, 1 cup	1.0 g

Adapted from USDA National Nutrient Database for Standard Reference Legacy.[16]

carbohydrate is high.[2] As with general health and nutrition, unsaturated fats from plant oils, nuts and seeds, and fatty fish are health-promoting and are recommended. Omega-3 fatty acids are of particular interest because of their impact on reducing inflammation and their role in optimizing brain health. Limiting saturated fat from meat products is key when developing a well-balanced meal plan. This includes limiting red meat, processed meat products, and full-fat dairy.

High-fat, low-carbohydrate diets are popular among endurance athletes. Fat is a source of energy in the form of circulating free fatty acids, intramuscular triglycerides, and adipose tissue. Fat is stored in the body, providing thousands of calories of energy that can be used during training.[25] Endurance athletes may try to become fat-adapted, using fat as their preferential energy source, to avoid "hitting the wall" or "bonking." This refers to the depletion of glycogen during endurance training.[26] Although a high-fat diet seems like a logical solution, exercising muscle during endurance sports will still need a supply of carbohydrate to keep up with the demand for ATP in addition to fat.[26] Triglycerides have the highest yield of ATP, but their rate of ATP turnover is low.[2] Glycogen produces higher muscle power and allows for sustained higher intensity paces during marathons.[11] Research on high-fat, low-carbohydrate diets for endurance sports lacks population size, robust evidence on performance enhancement, and has overall limited findings.[25]

Hydration

The human body is 50% to 70% water, with 65% in the intracellular spaces and 35% in the extracellular spaces.[27] Achieving euhydration, or optimal hydration, is essential for performance. Exercise can cause changes to the balance of fluids via sweat losses, respiration, and urine.[18,27] Exercise intensity can delay gastric emptying, affecting the absorption of fluid.[27] This occurs at high intensities, greater than 70% of Vo_{2max}.[27] Athletes should begin training in a state of euhydration and continue to replace fluids to avoid body mass losses greater than 2%, where decrements in performance are noted.[18] Avoiding overhydration, which can result in hyponatremia, is also a hydration goal.

Field testing an athlete's body mass changes is the most practical way to assess fluid losses. This involves calculating fluid losses per hour in body mass, known as an athlete's "sweat rate," and includes pretraining and posttraining body weight measurements while accounting for fluid intake and urinary losses during training. Other methods include urine specific gravity, urine color, and thirst. Urinary osmolality of greater than 900 mOsmol/kg reflects hypohydration, and less than 700 mOsmol/kg reflects euhydration.[18]

Hydration needs are unique to other nutrient needs. They are individualized depending on an athlete's sweat rate, exercise mode and intensity, duration of training, environmental conditions, equipment and uniform, and availability of fluid and fuel during training.[27] The longer and higher intensity an athlete trains, the higher the potential sweat rate. Athletes who perform in hot, humid climates are at higher risk for dehydration.[2,27,28] Hot and humid conditions can increase sweat losses and increase the risk for decreased blood flow to the brain and venous pooling, which can lead to syncope and heat exhaustion.[28] In addition, the material and weight of uniforms and equipment worn can impact sweat rate, as in the case for football players who sport heavy uniforms and often perform in the heat.[27]

Dehydration can pose a threat to the performance and health of the athlete, impacting blood volume, blood pressure, nervous system activity, and renal function.[29,30] The nervous and endocrine systems regulate hydration by affecting plasma osmolality and vascular volume.[29] As blood volume drops, the autonomic nervous system and

Table 6
Sample meal plan for a 66 kg female soccer athlete, training hard for 2 h 6x/week

Breakfast (7:30 AM)	Pretraining (9:30)	Intra-training (10:15–12:15)	Posttraining (12:45)	Lunch (2 PM)	Snack (5 PM)	Dinner (7:30 PM)
2 eggs	1 medium Banana	16 ounces sports drink	20 g protein shake	3 oz seasoned	5 oz cup vanilla	3 oz baked salmon
1.5 cups oatmeal	8 ounces sports		1 granola bar	roasted chicken	non-fat Greek	season with turmeric
with cinnamon	drink			1.5 cups rice and	yogurt	1.5 cups roasted
2 tsp honey				beans	½ cup berries	potatoes in olive oil
½ cup raspberries				1 cup sauteed	2 tbsp slivered	15 asparagus spears
8 oz orange juice				zucchini in	almond	
				garlic		

Calories: 2700.
Protein: 150 g
Carbohydrates: 400 g
Fat: 70 g fat.

endocrine system respond to increase plasma blood volume.[29] These changes can cause decrements in cognitive performance via decreased cerebral blood flow, decreased brain volume, and increased blood–brain barrier permeability.[30] Researchers have proposed that symptoms of hypohydration such as thirst, headaches, and fatigue may impact cognitive performance over physiologic effects.[30] In addition, there is individual variability in resiliency and the ability to overcome the effects of hypohydration.[30]

Hypohydration impacts physical performance by decreased blood flow to muscles, decreased blood volume, and hyperthermia, impacting muscle power, endurance, aerobic performance, and speed.[30] Endurance sports are more prone to hypohydration and decreased performance due to the duration of training. Losses of 2% to 7% body mass have been shown in cycling, marathon, and triathlon races.[31] Altered muscle energy metabolism can occur, causing increased lactate, glycogenolysis, and carbohydrate oxidation.[30] Hypohydration can induce hyperthermia, causing increased core body temperature and central nervous system fatigue.[30] This has been shown to impact sprint performance and decrease the ability to sustain maximal muscle activation.[30] It is important to note that increased core body temperature has been shown to improve sprint performance, but only during euhydration.[30]

A hydration strategy should include fluids throughout the day, during, and posttraining. The solution should contain a combination of glucose and fructose as well as sodium to optimize absorption and sustain energy output.[31] Sodium is the primary electrolyte lost and should be a focus during rehydration.[28,31] Plain water is ineffective at maintaining fluid balance during recovery, but can be used to rehydrate if consumed with a meal.[28] Athletes should consume 2 to 4 mL per pound 2 to 4 hours before training.[18] Although sweat rates vary, 0.4 to 0.8 L per hour of fluid is a general recommendation and should be adjusted for individual needs.[17] Posttraining 0.5 to 0.7 L of fluid should be consumed for every pound lost to account for urinary losses during rehydration.[18] Athletes should continue to consume fluids, including water, throughout the day to ensure their needs are met.

Nutrient Timing

The specific timing of meals, hydration, supplements, and snacks are essential to the success of an athlete's performance. The role of the sports dietitian is to translate this into food and supplement protocols for the athlete to follow and consume. **Table 6** provides an example of a meal plan demonstrating how the recommendations previously discussed can be strategically implemented for an athlete to obtain adequate nutrition for performance.

SUMMARY

Athletes' performance, health, and longevity in sports require specific attention to nutrition. When following an individualized plan, nutrition can amplify an athlete's ability to achieve higher performance levels. Specific focus on nutrient timing of proteins, carbohydrates, and fats is key to successfully restoring glycogen stores, repairing muscle, reducing exercise-induced inflammation, and promoting recovery.

The foundation of a successful sports nutrition plan includes adequate energy, carbohydrates, protein, fat, and fluids. Carbohydrate needs range from 3 to 12 g/kg/d depending on the duration and intensity of training.[7] Being the primary source of fuel, carbohydrates are needed throughout the day, before and after training, and during training when appropriate. Athletes' protein needs are higher than the current dietary recommendations of 0.8 g/kg per day and range from 1.2 to 2.0 g/kg/d.[2] This ensures an adequate amino acid pool is available, including enough leucine, to promote MPS and recovery. As for fat, the general recommendation is 1 g/kg/d to ensure essential fatty acids are obtained.[2] Supplementation of omega-3 fatty acids may be necessary. Hydration strategies should be tailored to the individual's specific sweat rate and sodium needs, including fluid throughout the day, during, and posttraining, as dehydration threatens cognitive and physical performance.

CLINICS CARE POINTS

- An athlete's total daily energy expenditure is often double their resting metabolic rate. Ensuring adequate calories are consumed is important to avoid low energy availability; therefore, referring competitive athletes to a registered dietitian nutritionist specializing in sports, preferably a Certified Specialist in Sports Dietetics, is vital to their performance and overall health.

- An athlete's primary fuel source is carbohydrates, especially at intensities greater than 60% Vo_{2max}. Athletes' needs range from 3 to 12 g/kg of carbohydrates per day, depending on the intensity and duration of training.

- Protein is essential for building and maintaining skeletal muscle in athletes. A range of 1.2 to 2.0 g/kg should be considered for this population. Excess protein is not recommended or needed to facilitate muscle growth or maintenance.

- Fat is essential and is a fuel source at rest and at low physical activity levels. Consumption of fats at 1.0 g/kg per day is recommended. High-fat, low-carbohydrate diets for endurance athletes are not recommended due to their high need for carbohydrates.

- Hydration needs are highly individual and depend on an athlete's sweat rate, training environment, intensity and duration of the training, and other factors such as their uniform. It is recommended that athletes start training euhydrated and continue with hydration during training. Beverages with sodium, glucose, and fructose are best for absorption and rehydration.

CONTRIBUTORS

A note of appreciation to Christina Chagris and Amber Palacios from the Long Island University Dietetic Internship program for their contributions to reviewing the research for this article.

DISCLOSURE

The author has nothing to disclose.

REFERENCES

1. Gastin PB. Energy system interaction and relative contribution during maximal exercise. Sports Med 2001;31(10):725–41.
2. Karpinski C, Rosenbloom C. Sports Nutrition: A Handbook for Professionals. Acad Nutr Diet 2017;6.
3. Mountjoy M, Sundgot-Borgen JK, Burke LM, et al. IOC consensus statement on relative energy deficiency in sport (RED-S): 2018 update. Br J Sports Med 2018;52:687–97.
4. Swanwick E, Matthews M. Energy systems: a new look at aerobic metabolism in stressful exercise. MOJ Sports Med 2018;2(1):15–22.

5. Smith-Ryan AE, Hirsch KR, Saylor HE, et al. Nutritional Considerations and Strategies to Facilitate Injury Recovery and Rehabilitation. J Athl Train 2020;55(9): 918–30.

6. Mehta J, Thompson B, Kling JM. The female athlete triad: It takes a team. Cleve Clin J Med 2018;85(4):313–20.

7. Reale R, Slater G, Burke LM. Acute-Weight-Loss Strategies for Combat Sports and Applications to Olympic Success. Int J Sports Physiol Perform 2017;12(2): 142–51.

8. Silvestre R, West C, Maresh CM, et al. Body composition and physical performance in men's soccer: a study of a National Collegiate Athletic Association Division I team. J Strength Cond Res 2006;20(1):177–83.

9. Ćopić N, Dopsaj M, Ivanović J, et al. Body composition and muscle strength predictors of jumping performance: differences between elite female volleyball competitors and nontrained individuals. J Strength Cond Res 2014;28(10):2709–16.

10. Silva MR, Paiva T. Poor precompetitive sleep habits, nutrients' deficiencies, inappropriate body composition and athletic performance in elite gymnasts. Eur J Sport Sci 2016;16(6):726–35.

11. Murray B, Rosenbloom C. Fundamentals of glycogen metabolism for coaches and athletes. Nutr Rev 2018;76(4):243–59.

12. Ormsbee MJ, Bach CW, Baur DA. Pre-exercise nutrition: the role of macronutrients, modified starches and supplements on metabolism and endurance performance. Nutrients 2014;6(5):1782–808. Published 2014 Apr 29.

13. Burke LM, Hawley JA, Wong SH, et al. Carbohydrates for training and competition. J Sports Sci 2011;29(Suppl 1):S17–27.

14. Volpe Stella Lucia. Glycemic Index and Athletic Performance. ACSM's Health Fitness J January 2011;15(1):32–3.

15. Jamurtas AZ, Tofas T, Fatouros I, et al. The effects of low and high glycemic index foods on exercise performance and beta-endorphin responses. J Int Soc Sports Nutr 2011;8:15. https://doi.org/10.1186/1550-2783-8-15.

16. Nutrients: Carbohydrate, by difference(g) - nal.usda.gov. Available at: https://www.nal.usda.gov/legacy/sites/default/files/carbohydrate.pdf. Accessed January 31, 2022.

17. Burke LM, van Loon LJC, Hawley JA. Postexercise muscle glycogen resynthesis in humans. J Appl Physiol (1985) 2017;122(5):1055–67.

18. Thomas DT, Erdman KA, Burke LM. Position of the Academy of Nutrition and Dietetics, Dietitians of Canada, and the American College of Sports Medicine: Nutrition and Athletic Performance. J Acad Nutr Diet 2016;116(3):501–28, published correction appears in J Acad Nutr Diet. 2017 Jan;117(1):146.

19. Areta JL, Burke LM, Ross ML, et al. Timing and distribution of protein ingestion during prolonged recovery from resistance exercise alters myofibrillar protein synthesis. J Physiol 2013;591(9):2319–31.

20. Moore Daniel R, Robinson Meghann J, Fry Jessica L, et al. Ingested protein dose response of muscle and albumin protein synthesis after resistance exercise in young men. Am J Clin Nutr 2009;89(1):161–8.

21. Mazzulla M, Volterman KA, Packer JE, et al. Whole-body net protein balance plateaus in response to increasing protein intakes during post-exercise recovery in adults and adolescents. Nutr Metab (Lond) 2018;15(62). https://doi.org/10.1186/s12986-018-0301-z.

22. Moore DR, Robinson MJ, Fry JL, et al. Ingested protein dose response of muscle and albumin protein synthesis after resistance exercise in young men. Am J Clin Nutr 2009;89(1):161–8.

23. van Vliet Stephan, Burd Nicholas A. The Skeletal Muscle Anabolic Response to Plant- versus Animal-Based Protein Consumption. J Nutr 2015;145(Issue 9): 1981–91.
24. Gorissen SHM, Crombag JJR, Senden JMG, et al. Protein content and amino acid composition of commercially available plant-based protein isolates. Amino Acids 2018;50:1685–95.
25. Bailey CP, Hennessy E. A review of the ketogenic diet for endurance athletes: performance enhancer or placebo effect? J Int Soc Sports Nutr 2020;17:33. https://doi.org/10.1186/s12970-020-00362-9.
26. Ipata P, Balestri F, Pesi R. The metabolic response of glycogen and free fatty acids to endurance exercise. Curr Metabolomics 2017;5(1):68–75.
27. Belval LN, Hosokawa Y, Casa DJ, et al. Practical Hydration Solutions for Sports. Nutrients 2019;11(7):1550.
28. Evans GH, James LJ, Shirreffs SM, et al. Optimizing the restoration and maintenance of fluid balance after exercise-induced dehydration. J Appl Physiol (1985) 2017;122(4):945–51.
29. Baker LB, Jeukendrup AE. Optimal composition of fluid-replacement beverages. Compr Physiol 2014;4(2):575–620.
30. Nuccio RP, Barnes KA, Carter JM, et al. Fluid Balance in Team Sport Athletes and the Effect of Hypohydration on Cognitive, Technical, and Physical Performance. Sports Med 2017;47(10):1951–82.
31. Orrù S, Imperlini E, Nigro E, et al. Role of Functional Beverages on Sport Performance and Recovery. Nutrients 2018;10(10):1470.

Nutrition for the Athlete
Beyond the Basics

Gabriela Barreto, MS, RD, CDN, CSSD*

KEYWORDS

- Sports nutrition • Supplements • Creatine • Injury recovery
- Relative energy deficiency in sports • Eating disorders • Female athlete triad

KEY POINTS

- Dietary sports supplementation can give athletes an edge in performance, adaptations, and recovery from training. Strong evidence exists for creatine, caffeine, nitric oxide, and omega-3 fatty acids.
- Injury recovery should be focused on preserving skeletal muscle and reducing inflammation through dietary interventions, including omega-3 fatty acids and creatine supplementation.
- Relative energy deficiency in sport results from low energy availability with concerns for menstrual, bone, and cardiovascular health, as well as performance markers.
- Eating disorders occur at higher rates in athletes compared with the general population. Careful monitoring, screening, and protocols should be instituted to protect an athlete's health.

INTRODUCTION

Athletes perform at high levels of competition and seek a competitive edge through training, nutrition, and recovery. Owing to this demand, dietary sports supplements may be beneficial for success. Of particular interest are caffeine, creatine, omega-3 fatty acids, and nitric oxide activators.[1–8] These supplements are well studied to be advantageous for performance, adaptations, and recovery. Creatine is the most well-studied supplement, benefiting muscle strength and power, glycogen replenishment, anaerobic training, and injury recovery.[1–3]

Athletes are prone to various injuries, related surgeries, and head trauma. Nutrition plays a role in preserving skeletal muscle and reducing inflammation through dietary interventions.[7–12] Increased energy needs are noted due to higher metabolic demands for recovery, even while immobilized.[7] Protein needs are also increased to minimize muscle mass losses.[7] Supplementation of creatine and omega-3s may also aid in

Staint Joseph's College, Brooklyn Campus, 245 Clinton Avenue, Brooklyn, NY 11205, USA
* Corresponding author
E-mail address: nutritionbygabby@gmail.com

Physician Assist Clin 7 (2022) 741–750
https://doi.org/10.1016/j.cpha.2022.06.005
2405-7991/22/© 2022 Elsevier Inc. All rights reserved.

recovery, muscle mass preservation, and modulating the inflammatory processes associated with injury.[7,8,11]

As discussed in the paper titled, *Nutrition for the Athlete: A Foundation for Success*, meeting an athlete's energy needs through properly distributed proteins, carbohydrates, and fats, as well as hydration and fluid intake, sets their nutrition foundation. The most important factor in an athlete's nutrition plan is having adequate energy availability. Low energy availability (LEA) leaves athletes with inadequate energy for metabolic processes and poses health and performance consequences. The negative consequences include, but are not limited to, menstrual, bone, cardiovascular health, and decreased performance markers.[13,14] This can lead to relative energy deficiency in sport (RED-S), a syndrome noted by a host of physiologic and performance detriments.[14]

This article will expand beyond the basics and provide an understanding of athletes' unique needs related to their health and performance. Discussion of the risk factors, screening, assessment, and treatment of RED-S and eating disorders (ED) will be reviewed. The role of supplementation, in addition to safe sources and dosage recommendations, in performance and injury recovery will be outlined to provide evidence-based recommendations for athletes.

DISCUSSION
Supplements

Ergogenic aids are supplements that claim to enhance the performance of athletes. They are used to enhance recovery; improve strength, speed, and endurance; reduce time to fatigue; and increase energy to give athletes a competitive advantage. Supplements well studied for athletes include creatine, caffeine, nitrates, and omega-3s.[1–6] Micronutrients of concern for athletes include iron and vitamin D.[3,6] Whereas whole foods are preferred for athletes to obtain nutrition, supplements play a role in enhancing the health and performance of the athlete.

Creatine

Creatine is the most well studied, effective, and safe supplement for athletes. Creatine supplementation can improve strength and muscle mass, glycogen stores, recovery, aerobic capacity, anaerobic threshold, sprint performance, and training tolerance.[1,2] Creatine is also helpful in recovery from injury, concussions, and cognitive health.[2] As discussed in the aforementioned companion paper, the phosphocreatine system provides a short energy supply intended for explosive power movements. Sports that may benefit from creatine supplementation are noted in **Box 1**.

Diets, including meat and poultry will contain about 1 to 2 g of creatine a day which saturates muscle creatine stores to 60% to 80%.[2] Vegetarian or vegan athletes who

---

Box 1
Sports enhanced by creatine[1]

Sports where creatine may enhance performance
   American football and powerlifting
   Olympic weightlifting, track and field events, and basketball
   Soccer
   American football and tennis
   Combat sports (ie, boxing, wrestling, and Muay Thai)
   Swim events (100 m, 200 m)
   Track events (400 m, 800 m)

rely on plant-based protein sources have lower creatine levels, and supplementation can increase intramuscular creatine stores.[2] Typically, when an athlete takes creatine, there is a loading phase followed by a maintenance phase. Loading phases in the literature that have shown to increase intramuscular phosphocreatine (PCr) stores rapidly include 0.3 g/kg/d for 3 to 5 days or 20 g/d for 5 to 7 days.[1,2] A maintenance dosage of 3 to 5 g/d to maintain PCr stores is recommended.[1,3] Additionally, consumption of a mixed protein and carbohydrate meal with ~50 g of each can increase creatine absorption through the insulin response to the meal.[3]

Caffeine

Caffeine is a well-established supplement used widely in the athletic and general population. It aids in increasing endorphins, improves alertness and response, decreases the perception of exercise exertion, and improves neuromuscular function.[3] Regarding performance, caffeine has been shown to increase endurance capacity, such as time to fatigue, improve time trial performance in cycling, and improve sprint performance and repeat sprint performance during intermittent sports (ie, soccer).[3] The literature recommends 3 to 6 mg/kg of caffeine in an anhydrous or pill form 60 minutes before training.[3] Lower doses of caffeine, 100 to 300 mg, may also affect endurance performance if consumed 15 to 80 minutes into exercise.[3] It is important to note that the National Collegiate Athletic Association (NCAA) bans caffeine supplements at the collegiate level.

Nitrates

Dietary nitrates are found naturally occurring in foods, such as beets and spinach. Nitrate consumption increases the availability of nitric oxide, converted via bacteria in the mouth and during digestion.[4] Nitric oxide aids in vasodilation, cellular respiration, and angiogenesis.[5] This function of nitric oxide enhances performance by increasing nutrient and oxygen delivery to cells, increasing clearance of metabolic by-products from high-intensity exercise (ie, lactic acid), decreasing adenosine triphosphate (ATP) consumption in exercising muscle, and decreasing oxygen consumption during exercise.[5] These affect performance markers by increasing time to exhaustion, decreasing oxygen cost of exercise, lowering blood pressure, and increasing exercise capacity.[3,4,6] These effects have been observed for training lasting 5 to 30 minutes, with limited evidence of benefits observed during training greater than 40 minutes.[6]

Supplementation protocols suggest 5 to 9 mmol (310–560 mg) of nitrate supplementation 2 to 3 hours before training.[3,4,6] Further benefits are seen when intake of nitrate supplementation is taken 3 days consecutively.[5] Athletes can meet this via 250 to 500 g of high nitrate vegetables (ie, beetroot, endive, fennel, lettuce, radish, rocket, and spinach).[5] A dietary supplement is a more accurate way to reach their needs as food content may vary.[5] Beetroot juice is the most common form of nitric oxide supplementation studied.

Micronutrients

Supplementation of micronutrients may be necessary. Iron is essential to form hemoglobin, deliver oxygen to muscles, and remove carbon dioxide. The potential for suboptimal iron stores is of concern for athletes. This is due to potential increased gastrointestinal blood losses, increased hepcidin from high-intensity exercise, footstrike hemolysis, and possible bursting of hepcidin blocking iron.[15] Vegetarian and vegan diets can pose another risk for iron deficiency, as nonheme sources of iron are as well absorbed. For athletes with inadequate iron status, greater than 18 mg/d for women and greater than 8 mg/d for men may be beneficial.[3] Higher doses for more severe iron deficiency should be under the care of a health care professional. Vitamin D deficiency is a common micronutrient deficiency in the general and athletic population. This is particularly of concern in the northern states because of the lack of ultraviolet B (UVB) rays in the fall and winter months. Insufficient or deficient vitamin D in an athlete may negatively impact bone health.[3] The recommended intake is 800 to2000 IU/d to maintain a healthy status.[3] A complete summary of supplement recommendations, dosing, and food sources is provided in **Table 1**.

It is important to note that The United States Food and Drug Administration does not regulate supplements, and at times banned substances have been found in nonbanned supplements for athletes.[16] This has resulted in athletes being disqualified from the competition, including the Olympic games.[16] Contamination can occur because of poor manufacturing processes or intentionally by unethical manufacturers.[16] The World Anti-Doping Association and the NCAA regulate the usage and banning of substances for athletes at professional and collegiate levels. The importance of adherence to banned substances by these organizations is crucial for an athlete's career, as these organizations routinely test athletes. Clinicians can visit each organization's web site as banned substances differ for collegiate and professional sports.

Athletes should be aware and educated on identifying safe sources of supplements. Athletes should be guided to seek supplements certified by third-party testing organizations, such as NSF Certified for Sport, Informed Choice Sport, Consumer Labs and USP Dietary Supplement Certified. See **Fig. 1** for identifying labels.

Nutrition for Injury Recovery

An adequate and balanced diet is necessary for the prevention of injury as well as for recovery and rehabilitation. When an injury occurs, an athlete's resting metabolic rate (RMR) may increase to meet the energy demand of cellular turnover.[9] This may increase by 20% for a minor injury to up to 100% of their RMR for major surgery or an injury like a burn.[9] To determine an athlete's energy needs, the RMR is multiplied by a corresponding activity factor and a stress factor. Stress factors related to the injury are listed in **Table 2**. This will account for the energy needed for repair depending on the level of injury.[9]

Energy needs during injury = RMR × Activity Factor × Stress Factor[7]

The major considerations in injury nutrition are muscle atrophy, decreased muscle protein synthesis (MPS), loss of strength, and proteolysis.[7] It is vital in recovery from injury to maintain energy balance via adequate nutrition intake to prevent muscle loss from disuse or immobility.[9] Muscle disuse atrophy rapidly occurs at a rate of 0.5% per day, and one can lose 150–400 g of muscle tissue in the first 1–2 weeks.[9] Energy intakes of 25–30 cal/kg of body weight, which have been shown to fight sarcopenia, are recommended.[9] Carbohydrates remain a main source of energy and are required at a rate of 3–5 g/kg depending on injury, activity, and overall energy needs.[7]

As noted earlier, MPS is stimulated by mechanical damage to the muscle as well as adequate intake of protein and the amino acid leucine. Higher protein needs are warranted in recovery, as MPS may be blunted, at 1.6–2.5 g/kg.[10] Protein, with adequate leucine content, in amounts of 20–40 g should be consumed every 3–4 hours. This should be high-quality, quickly digested protein. Casein may be helpful before sleep.

Fat is necessary for energy and cell proliferation. An important type of fat in injury recovery is the omega-3 fatty acids for their role as an anti-inflammatory agent. Supplementing with 2000–4000 mg may reduce inflammation and maximize protein synthesis.[7] Omega-3 fatty acids are long-chain fatty acids known as eicosapentaenoic acid (EPA) and docosahexaenoic acid (DHA). DHA is the useable form of omega-3, and EPA is converted well to DHA in the body. Alpha-linolenic acid (ALA) is a form

Table 1
Supplement recommendations

Supplements	Dosages	Impact on Performance	Food Sources
Creatine	*Loading:* 0.3 g/kg/d for 3–5 d OR 20 g for 5–7 d[1,2] *Maintenance Dose* 3–5 g/d[1,3]	↑ Muscle strength and hypertrophy[1,2] ↑ Glycogen stores[1,2] ↑ Recovery[1,2] ↑ Aerobic capacity[1,2] ↑ Anaerobic threshold[1,2] ↑ Sprint performance[1,2] ↑ Training tolerance[1,2]	Meats, fish, and poultry
Caffeine	3–6 mg/kg 60 minutes prior to exercise in anhydrous or pill form[3] Low doses at <3 g/kg or ~ 200 mg pretraining with carbohydrate source[3]	↑ Endurance capacity[3] ↑ Sprint performance[3] ↑ Time trial performance in endurance sports[3]	Coffee, tea, and sodas
Nitrates	5–9 mmol (310–560 mg) of nitrate supplementation 2–3 hours before training[3,4,6] Potential benefit to 3 d consecutive before performance[5]	↑ Time to exhaustion[3,4,6] ↓ Oxygen cost of exercise[5] ↓ Blood pressure[3,4,6] ↑ Exercise capacity[5] ↓ ATP consumed by muscle[5] ↑ Clearance of metabolic by-products[5]	Beetroot, endive, fennel, lettuce, radish, rocket, and spinach
Omega-3	2000–4000 mg/d[7]	Reduce inflammation,[7] improve recovery time, maximize MPS,[7] recovery from mild TBI[8]	Salmon, tuna, mackerel, cod liver oil, herring, oysters, sardines, fortified milk, and eggs
Iron	15 mg/d 3		*Heme iron:* Meat, fish, poultry, sardines, and mussels *Nonheme:* Enriched cereals, beans, dried fruits, split peas, and enriched pasta
Vitamin D	800–2000 IU/d[3]		Cod liver oil, salmon, trout, UVB-exposed mushrooms, fortified milk, and eggs

Note: Omega-3 will be discussed in the section titled, "Nutrition for Injury Recovery."

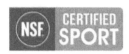

Fig. 1. Logos of the third-party testing organization.

of omega-3 found in nuts, seeds, and avocados. ALA is not as well converted to DHA in the body. Therefore, foods rich in DHA and EPA are important to consume, such as fatty fish and fortified milk.

Omega-3 has been studied for its anti-inflammatory properties and effects on oxidative stress and proinflammatory markers, such as cytokines.[11] Inflammation may play a role in muscle wasting, muscle signaling, muscle mass, and endurance, although the mechanism warrants more research.[9] Besides its anti-inflammatory properties, omega-3 fatty acids increase MPS through the hyperaminoacidemia–hyperinsulinemia response.[7] The anti-inflammatory effect of omega-3s causes an increase in blood flow, producing this increased MPS response.[7]

Creatine monohydrate is one of the most researched supplements in sports nutrition. Consuming creatine during immobilization from injury had favorable outcomes on muscle strength and lean mass, especially when combined with rehabilitation.[7] The recommended dosing is 5 g per day or loading of 20 g per day for 5 days by consuming four 5 g servings throughout the day.[7]

Concussions are a top concern for contact sports, such as football, soccer, rugby, and competitive cheerleading and dance. Considered a mild traumatic brain injury (TBI), concussions increase the brain's consumption and use of energy and nutrients.[12] It is important to note that most of the evidence for nutrition that is related to concussions has been provided by animal models. After a TBI, creatine is reduced, and its supplementation can aid in increasing ATP stores.[7] Large doses of 0.4 g/kg/ d post-TBI for 6 months improved cognitive function and decreased headaches, dizziness, and fatigue.[7]

Studies focus on supplementation to prevent or attenuate symptoms of concussions. After a concussion, DHA levels decrease in the brain.[8] Omega-3 fatty acid supplementation in the form of DHA has been shown to decrease injury to axons in the brain and markers of apoptosis.[8] DHA is particularly noted in brain health and postconcussion care as DHA constitutes 97% of omega-3s in the brain.[8] Estimates from animal studies suggest a dosage of 40 mg/kg/d, yet human clinical trials await more reliable recommendations.[8] The current recommendations for general health by organizations, such as the American Heart Association range from 250 to 500 mg/d.

Relative Energy Deficiency in Sport and Female Athlete Triad

As discussed in the aforementioned companion paper, LEA can affect an athlete's health and performance. The Female Athlete Triad was first established as remarkable

Table 2 Stress factors[7]	
Minor injury (ankle sprain, dislocation)	1.2
Minor surgery, clean wound, bone fracture	1.2
Infected wound	1.5
Major trauma (anterior cruciate ligament reconstruction surgery)	1.5
Severe burn	1.5

LEA symptoms coupled with menstrual dysfunction and decreased bone mineral density (BMD).[13] Adequate energy availability can be achieved at 45 cal/kg of fat-free mass (FFM).[13] LEA occurs at 30 cal/kg of FFM, leading to disruption in BMD and menstrual dysfunction in females.[13] In males, low testosterone, hormonal disruptions, and low BMD can also occur at LEA.[13] As male athletes also experience such symptoms, RED-S has been adopted in recent literature to discuss these complexities.[14] **Table 3** highlights the potential consequences of LEA and RED-S in athletes.

Several risk factors exist in the development of RED-S. Sports emphasizing leanness, endurance, weight class, and esthetics are at higher risk for developing the female athlete triad.[13] Athletes with histories of ED and disordered eating (DE) are at higher risk.[13,14] Whereas these place athletes at higher risk, LEA can occur without DE, ED, and outside weight class sports.[17] Athletes may receive misinformation on nutrition and how to decrease body fat or have a lack of time and/or resources to meet their high energy needs.[17]

An interdisciplinary team approach is necessary, including medical, nutritional, psychological, coaching, and training staff. Deciding whether an athlete is fit to remain in play is to be made by collaboration between all team members. If an athlete is taken out of a play, a return to play plan focuses on restoring the athlete's physical and psychological health.[18] The return to play and treatment outlined by De Souza and colleagues[18] in their treatment and return to play consensus provides a detailed outline for practitioners to use as a reference.

EATING DISORDERS IN ATHLETES

High-performing athletes are at a greater risk of developing DE and ED.[17] Studies have shown that 6%–50% of female and 0%–19% of male athletes suffer from DE or ED.[17,19] ED is an umbrella term for numerous diagnosable illnesses related to eating behavior. Refer to the *Diagnostic Statistical Manual of Mental Disorders*, Fifth Edition (DSM-V) for a complete source on ED.

Eating behaviors range from optimal nutrition to DE to ED. Optimal nutrition is defined as individual nutrition practices that support the athlete's health, energy, and performance needs.[17] DE is defined as engaging in restrictive eating, such as skipping meals or food groups, compulsive eating or exercise, and restriction of calories without meeting the DSM-V criteria for an ED.[17] DE can also include restrictive fad diets that involve energy restriction, binge eating, use of laxatives and diuretics, vomiting, diet pills, and/or excessive training.[17] An ED is a diagnosable mental illness

Table 3	
Health and performance consequences[14]	
Health Consequences	**Performance Consequences**
Metabolic disturbances	↓ Muscle strength
Impaired immune function	↓ Glycogen stores
Endocrine impairment	↓ Cognitive performance
Menstrual dysfunction	Impaired training response
↓ Bone health	↓ Cardiovascular health and endurance
Impaired growth and development	Mental health decline (ie, depression)
Gastrointestinal disturbances	
Hematological impairments	

meeting the criteria found in the DSM-V. An individual can fluctuate between optimal nutrition, DE, and ED at any point, as those in recovery from DE/ED can have relapses.

There are numerous risk factors in an athlete's development of an ED. Psychological risk factors, such as anxiety, depression, high-stress reactivity, poor self-esteem, distorted body image, and history of trauma place an individual at higher risk.[17] Additional risk factors include social media use, societal ideal body image, peer pressure, life transitions, co-morbidities, such as celiac or gastrointestinal disorders, and weight-based teasing.[17]

Sports-specific risk factors can promote DE/ED behaviors. When body shape and size are linked to the sport's success, a higher likelihood of DE/ED symptoms can arise. The sports community may normalize DE and reinforce unhealthy eating habits, especially in sports where low body fat or a thin body shape is encouraged.[19] Certain body ideals are promoted, such as thinness in long-distance runners and promoting DE behaviors.[17] Additionally, muscle dysmorphia, giving men the pressure to look more muscular, can increase the risk for DE/ED.[20]

Recognizing and appropriate treatment for DE/ED is an essential part of the role of the health care professionals, coaching, and training staff. The gold standard for ED assessment and screening is *The Eating Disorder Assessment Examination 17.0* T (EDE 17.0).[17] Once an individual is screened and suspected of DE or ED, a multidisciplinary team approach is needed, including medical, psychological, and nutrition professionals who specialize in ED treatment.[17] Any athlete presenting with stress fractures and/or menstrual dysfunction should be screened for RED-S and DE/ED.[17] The dietitian will play a significant role in helping the athlete meet their energy needs and re-establish normal menstrual function through adequate nutrition and weight restoration if needed. The medical team plays a crucial role in monitoring laboratories, cardiac health, bone health, and having a protocol for medical clearance for return to play. In this decision-making process, a team approach should be taken, including coaching and training staff.

SUMMARY

Athletes' performance, health, and longevity in sports require specific attention to nutrition. Tailored nutrition practices can be advantageous to a performance by consuming adequate energy, macronutrients, and micronutrients. As athletes' bodies perform at higher levels of physical demand, supplementation to aid in performance, health, and injury recovery may be beneficial. Ergogenic aids, such as creatine, caffeine, and dietary nitrates may enhance multiple performance factors.[3] During injury and concussion recovery, athletes may benefit from omega-3 and creatine supplementation.[7,9,11] Supplement safety is vital as banned substances can be found in approved supplements. Athletes should be guided to choose supplements tested by third-party companies.

Without adequate nutrition, athletes can experience LEA that can result in RED-S, causing harm to health and performance.[13,14] Focusing on weight and body composition is also high risk, as athletes are more prone to DE/ED.[17] A performance-first approach should be taken when discussing food, weight, and body composition to reinforce the role of nutrition in an athlete's career. Screening athletes who present with risk factors related to DE/ED can help identify athletes and provide proper treatment and counseling. Within the school, collegiate, and professional setting, protocols should be established to help identify, treat, and return athletes to play when recovering from DE/ED and RED-S. Professional guidance from the medical, nutrition, and performance teams is essential in ensuring an athlete's success on and off the field.

CLINICS CARE POINTS

- An athlete's sport, position, and volume of training may warrant the use of supplementation. Evidence-based supplementation recommendations should be used to enhance performance, health, and recovery.
- Supplements should be chosen from a brand that participates in third-party testing, such as the NSF Certified for Sport, Informed Choice Sport, Consumer Labs and USP Dietary Supplement Certified.
- During injury, the major role of nutrition is to minimize muscle loss, attenuate inflammation, and aid in recovery. Metabolic rate and energy needs increase in response to injury, despite immobilization. Increased energy intake, higher protein intake between 1.6 and 2.5 g/kg/d, and supplementation with creatine and omega-3 fatty acids may be warranted.
- Relative energy deficiency in sport requires screening and intervention from an interdisciplinary team. During the treatment of athletes, screening for the noted health and physical consequences is of importance. Having treatment and return to play protocols in practice and within organizations is recommended.
- Higher rates of eating disorders and disordered eating are seen among an athletic population, particularly in weight-based and esthetic-based sports. Using *The Eating Disorder Assessment Examination 17.0* assessment tool on athletes with potential risk is the key. Having a network of professionals who specialize in eating disorder treatment for athletes is suggested.

DISCLOSURE

The author has nothing to disclose.

REFERENCES

1. Buford TW, Kreider RB, Stout JR, et al. International Society of Sports Nutrition position stand: creatine supplementation and exercise. J Int Soc Sports Nutr 2007; 4(6). https://doi.org/10.1186/1550-2783-4-6.
2. Wax B, Kerksick CM, Jagim AR, et al. Creatine for Exercise and Sports Performance, with Recovery Considerations for Healthy Populations. Nutrients 2021; 13(6):1915.
3. Maughan RJ, Burke LM, Dvorak J, et al. IOC consensus statement: dietary supplements and the high-performance athlete. Br J Sports Med 2018;52(7):439–55.
4. Peeling P, Binnie MJ, Goods PSR, et al. Evidence-Based Supplements for the Enhancement of Athletic Performance. Int J Sport Nutr Exerc Metab 2018; 28(2):178–87.
5. Macuh M, Knap B. Effects of Nitrate Supplementation on Exercise Performance in Humans: A Narrative Review. Nutrients 2021;13(9):3183.
6. Jones AM. Dietary Nitrate Supplementation and Exercise Performance. Sports Med 2014;44:35–45.
7. Smith-Ryan AE, Hirsch KR, Saylor HE, et al. Nutritional Considerations and Strategies to Facilitate Injury Recovery and Rehabilitation. J Athl Train 2020;55(9): 918–30.
8. Barrett EC, McBurney MI, Ciappio ED. Ω-3 fatty acid supplementation as a potential therapeutic aid for the recovery from mild traumatic brain injury/concussion1,2. Adv Nutr 2014;5(3):268–77.
9. Papadopoulou SK. Rehabilitation Nutrition for Injury Recovery of Athletes: The Role of Macronutrient Intake. Nutrients 2020;12(8):2449.

10. Wall BT, Morton JP, van Loon LJ. Strategies to maintain skeletal muscle mass in the injured athlete: nutritional considerations and exercise mimetics. Eur J Sport Sci 2015;15(1):53–62.
11. Calder PC, Albers R, Antoine JM, et al. Inflammatory disease processes and interactions with nutrition. Br J Nutr 2009;101(Suppl 1):S1–45.
12. Walrand S, Gaulmin R, Aubin R, et al. Nutritional factors in sport- related concussion. Neurochirurgie 2021;67(3):255–8.
13. Weiss Kelly AK, Hecht S. COUNCIL ON SPORTS MEDICINE AND FITNESS. The Female Athlete Triad. Pediatrics 2016;138(2):e20160922.
14. Mountjoy M, Sundgot-Borgen JK, Burke LM, et al. IOC consensus statement on relative energy deficiency in sport (RED-S): 2018 update. Br J Sports Med 2018;52:687–97.
15. Clénin G, Cordes M, Huber A, et al. Iron deficiency in sports - definition, influence on performance and therapy. Swiss Med Wkly 2015;145:w14196.
16. Mathews NM. Prohibited Contaminants in Dietary Supplements. Sports Health 2018;10(1):19–30.
17. Wells KR, Jeacocke NA, Appaneal R, et al. The Australian Institute of Sport (AIS) and National Eating Disorders Collaboration (NEDC) position statement on disordered eating in high performance sport. Br J Sports Med 2020;54(21):1247–58.
18. De Souza MJ, Nattiv A, Joy E, et al. Female Athlete Triad Coalition Consensus Statement on Treatment and Return to Play of the Female Athlete Triad: 1st International Conference held in San Francisco, California, May 2012 and 2nd International Conference held in Indianapolis, Indiana, May 2013. Br J Sports Med 2014; 48(4):289.
19. Becker CB, McDaniel L, Bull S, et al. Can we reduce eating disorder risk factors in female college athletes? A randomized exploratory investigation of two peer-led interventions. Body Image 2012;9(1):31–42.
20. Leone JE, Sedory EJ, Gray KA. Recognition and treatment of muscle dysmorphia and related body image disorders. J Athl Train 2005;40(4):352–9 (47).

Moving?

Make sure your subscription moves with you!

To notify us of your new address, find your **Clinics Account Number** (located on your mailing label above your name), and contact customer service at:

Email: journalscustomerservice-usa@elsevier.com

800-654-2452 (subscribers in the U.S. & Canada)
314-447-8871 (subscribers outside of the U.S. & Canada)

Fax number: 314-447-8029

Elsevier Health Sciences Division
Subscription Customer Service
3251 Riverport Lane
Maryland Heights, MO 63043

*To ensure uninterrupted delivery of your subscription, please notify us at least 4 weeks in advance of move.

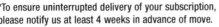